ABOUT EPILEPSY

DONALD SCOTT, MRCP DPM

ABOUT EPILEPSY

SECOND EDITION

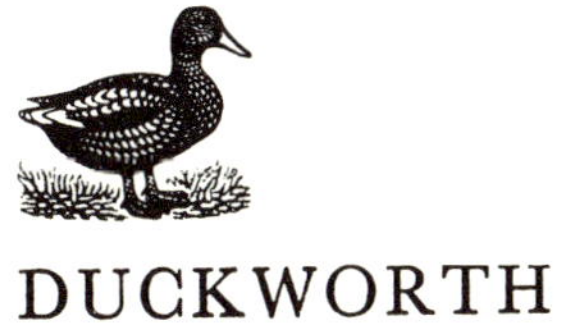

DUCKWORTH

First published in 1969 by
Gerald Duckworth & Co. Ltd,
The Old Piano Factory
43 Gloucester Crescent, London NW1

Second edition 1973

© *1969* DONALD F. SCOTT

SBN *7156 0438 4*

Printed Offset Litho in Great Britain by
Cox & Wyman Ltd
London, Fakenham and Reading

Contents

To A.M.S.

Preface to the revised edition

SINCE THIS book was first published in 1969, there have been
a number of changes in the care of the epileptic person, though
the basic problem of the causation of epilepsy remains. In
particular, more attention is now being paid to the social aspects
of epilepsy, and the multi-disciplinary approach is more common both in the United States and in Britain—where, however,
the full impact of the Government report "People with Epilepsy"
is still to be felt. I have described these changes of approach,
together with the results of many research studies, in chapter
XVII. Mention is also made of new neurosurgical techniques
which could prove of immense value in treatment. The
Bibliography has been enlarged, and minor corrections have
been made throughout the book to bring it into line with
changes in medical opinion.

I am grateful to many colleagues for suggestions incorporated
in this new edition, particularly to Dr Otto Magnus for his
detailed comments, and to Mrs Winifred Dawson, of the British
Epilepsy Association, who assisted especially in up-dating the
sections on social matters.

London   D.F.S.

February, 1973

Preface to the first edition

THIS BOOK aims to inform a wide range of people about epilepsy
and related conditions. At present there is no comprehensive,
non-technical yet up-to-date account, in a short compass, of the
many facets of epilepsy. In this book the medical, surgical and
social aspects, among many others, are discussed. Though
much is known about epilepsy, much still remains to be
clarified, hence an account of research in progress at present is
included.

The book is intended for those who will encounter epileptic

people professionally, such as nurses, social workers and teachers. In addition, it is hoped that students of medicine and of related fields will find it a valuable introduction to the subject; for these, particularly, a comprehensive bibliography is provided. Parents, relatives and the epileptic sufferers themselves will find information here which will be of value and interest. For them and the general public who may be unfamiliar with the terminology, a glossary of medical terms is included.

Secrecy and lack of information are two conditions which in the past have bred attitudes harmful to the epileptic person. If the present book helps the epileptic sufferer to lead a fuller and happier life, it will have amply fulfilled its purpose.

The author wishes to express his gratitude to many senior colleagues who have helped him to gain experience in this subject, particularly Dr M. Driver, Mr M. Falconer, Dr D. W. Liddell, Dr J. H. Margerison, and Professor D. Pond. Thanks are due to Mr G. Burden of the British Epilepsy Association for his constant help and encouragement. To him, to Dr J. H. Margerison and to Professor D. Pond grateful thanks, for careful reading of the whole manuscript and for helpful comment. The author is also particularly indebted to Mr David Sutherland Graeme for help with the historical, biographical and literary material, and to Dr C. Ounsted for help with the section on the inheritance of epilepsy.

Thanks are also due to Mrs D. Austin, Mrs C. Markham and Mrs J. Butcher for secretarial help at various stages of preparation of the manuscript, and to Dr P. Prior and Mr R. S. Ruddich, of the London Hospital, for help with the illustrations; also to the Pergamon Press who have kindly allowed the reproduction of figures 1, 3, 4, 5, 6, 7, 14 and 16.

Finally, the author wishes to thank the authors of many books and articles on the subject read over the past five years, who have contributed to ideas and opinions in this book, and the many colleagues, too numerous to name, who have helped in its preparation.

London   D.F.S.

April, 1969

CHAPTER ONE

Fits, faints and falls

A GUARDSMAN faints on parade; a housewife trips over the edge of a frayed stair carpet; both these events evoke sympathy and comment. A young man having a fit in the street, however, causes shock and perhaps revulsion in the passers-by. This reaction may be related to some atavistic fear of death or of being struck by an evil spirit; it is certainly not the response of a rational man. In fact, the fit is just as understandable as the other events, and in this case the sufferer deserves more sympathy than either the guardsman or the housewife. The fits will almost certainly recur, whereas the faint or the fall were only isolated incidents. The alliterative title of this chapter was chosen not to intrigue but to suggest at the same time the difficulties and the interesting individual aspects and relations of fits, faints and falls.

It is important for the doctor to decide which of these things happened in any given instance, before he begins to think about treatment. Almost everyone has had a fall or a faint at some time, and many could claim to have experienced a fit, if a "fit of temper" or a "fit of pique" are included under this name. But to the doctor "fit" has a more precise meaning; he applies it only to an epileptic fit. By "faint" the layman understands any brief, unpleasant sensation of complete weakness or collapse into unconsciousness, but to the doctor this event may indicate any one of several conditions. It sometimes occurs in those with heart disease. The heart may suddenly beat in too rapid and shallow a way, so that insufficient blood reaches the brain or, conversely, too slowly—with the same result. The onlooker who notices these faints may be surprised to see that the person who has fainted does not always recover at once. His limp state may change to one of rigid paralysis followed by a jerking attack. A faint due to heart disease has passed imperceptibly into a fit.

A "fall" is generally considered a harmless event. This may be so in the case of tripping over a carpet. But sometimes children who fall are found to have epilepsy, or middle-aged ladies fall and are found to be suffering from a disease of the arteries at the base of the brain.

Fits, faints and falls, then, are not the simple, separate events we usually suppose. All may occur on their own or in combination with each other, and all may be symptoms of epilepsy. To the layman the doctor's formula "epilepsy itself is not a disease but a symptom" is puzzling and needs some explanation. It mainly implies that epileptic attacks occur not just in one disease but in a variety of conditions. We have seen how easy it it is for an ordinary observer to mistake the significance of fits, faints and falls. Headaches and sickness are likewise symptoms, not diseases, and, as with fits, we must attempt to find the underlying cause. Sometimes a brain tumour or scar is the source of the trouble, but in other cases diagnosis is far more difficult, because no definite cause for the epilepsy can be found. Generalised disease may be present which affects the healthy brain indirectly through the circulation of the blood. This too leads to fits. Some of these conditions can be corrected and the fits controlled.

The contribution of Hippocrates

The twentieth century, with its technical advances, has brought new ideas and new tools to bear on the problems of fits, faints and falls. However, epilepsy was well known even to the ancients.

2

Hippocrates (460 to 377 BC), for instance, discusses it. Hippocrates was born on the Greek island of Cos, a medical centre for the ancient world. He considered that epilepsy was the result of brain disease and berated his colleagues who regarded it as some manifestation of divine intervention, maintaining that they said this merely to cloak their ignorance.

Hippocrates blamed imbalance of the four humours—blood, phlegm, yellow bile and black bile—as the cause of fits. This, as we now know, was a fallacious concept but at least it attempted to make epilepsy comprehensible on a rational basis, and placed the cause within the body, not outside it. By his accurate study of epileptic patients Hippocrates was able to put forward original views on the function of the brain:

> Man should be fully aware of the fact that it is from the brain and from the brain only that our feelings of joy, pleasure, of laughing arise as well as our sorrow, our pain, our grief and our tears. We are thinking with the brain and we can see and hear and we are able to draw distinction between ugliness and beauty, bad and good and what is pleasant and unpleasant.

In the dark and early Middle Ages other views on the causation of epilepsy were enunciated; there was a popular desire to connect it with supernatural powers, and this found its Christian counterpart in the association of epileptic sufferers with particular saints, notably St Valentine in Germany. Later, a popular view that epilepsy was contagious appeared to be held both by laymen and physicians alike. Since the breath was thought to be infectious it seemed logical to establish isolation hosptials for the epileptic patient, as was already being done for lepers.

In the sixteenth and seventeenth centuries demoniacal possession was of great interest to physicians, few of whom doubted the existence of Satan, who was believed to be in league with a host of devils. Epilepsy was thought to be the work of these malevolent creatures and this view, understandably, created certain problems of diagnosis and treatment! It was only when such physicians as Thomas Willis (1622–75), often called the founder of modern neurology, re-established the view of Hippocrates that epilepsy arose from diseases of the brain, that these irrational views were gradually superseded.

Another English physician, Hughlings Jackson (born 1835) advanced contemporary knowledge of epilepsy even further.(It is possible that his interest was stimulated by his wife's unusual form of epilepsy; this kind, which begins as a twitch in the big toe or thumb and spreads until the whole of the arm or leg is twitching, is now usually called Jacksonian epilepsy.) Hughlings Jackson was able by careful observation to define epilepsy as the "occasional, sudden, excessive, rapid and local discharges of grey matter". It was only much later, with the discovery by Hans Berger of the electro-encephalograph in the 1920s, that this view of epilepsy could be confirmed, as we shall see later.

How many people have epilepsy?

There has been, therefore, progress over the centuries in the study of epilepsy, though perhaps more emphasis has been placed on the condition of epilepsy than on the epileptic sufferer himself, who is still confronted with considerable difficulties. Epilepsy should be more widely understood, because a great number of people suffer from it; just how many is impossible to determine exactly because of different interpretations of the condition. Some may have only one attack in a lifetime, and these people should not really be included in the statistics. Again many who have had attacks will not reveal the fact even to their wives or doctors. Thus the figures sometimes given are bound to err; more often than not they are an underestimate. In the United States it has been suggested that as many as one in fifty of the population have had epileptic seizures at some time in their lives. To assess accurately just how many people do suffer from epilepsy and other diseases of the nervous system, a recent study, published in 1966, was carried out in the city of Carlisle. The records of hospitals and general practitioners were examined and, in addition, visits were made to a proportion of householders in an attempt to discover unrecorded instances of the disease. If the findings of this detailed study of a small section of the population can be taken as representative, then probably about 253,000 people in this country have epilepsy (0·5 per cent), and some 13,000 new cases of epilepsy occur every year (0·03 per cent). This compares with 53,000 people known to suffer from Parkinson's disease and 37,000 patients who have disseminated sclerosis. It has also been suggested that in the whole world some 32,000,000 people are suffering from epilepsy. Clearly, then, on a national or on an international basis this condition is of great importance.

What is epilepsy?

What then are the characteristics of those with epilepsy? The only thing that marks them out from their fellow human beings is the fact that they have fits. As will be seen later, their personalities, intelligence and abilities are as varied as those of persons free from fits. The word "epilepsy" itself needs explanation. It comes from a Greek word meaning "to seize" or "to halt", whereas "fit" is an English word which was not used with this meaning until the sixteenth century and which described then, as now, a transitory attack. "Epilepsy" is used for the condition in the brain, and "fits" to describe what the observer sees. Epilepsy, then, is a disorder of the brain which expresses itself briefly and repeatedly.

Fits vary in form from the commonest and most dramatic one, the convulsion, to the mild form, the almost unnoticed *petit mal* attacks. It is generally the convulsion, however, which claims attention. The great Roman poet Lucretius had obviously seen a convulsion and gives us his account:

> Oft, too, some wretch before our startled sight
> Struck as with lightning by some keen disease
> Drops sudden by the dread attack o'erpowered.
> He foams, he trembles and he faints.
> Now rigid, now convulsed, his labouring lungs heave
>   quick, quivers each exhausted limb. . . .

5

Fits, faints and falls

In contrast to this, the child in the classroom with the momentary vacant stare or fluttering eyelids has also had a fit. His *petit mal* has not even been seen by anyone, except perhaps by an observant teacher. In some fits the patient's awareness may be disturbed either to the point of unconsciousness, as in a convulsion, or partially, as in some forms of temporal lobe epilepsy. As a result, the memory may be impaired—even the child with the *petit mal* attack may lose his place when reading aloud.

In this book the following terms are used in a specific way. *Fit* is always used to indicate an epileptic phenomenon. It may mean a mild or severe epileptic attack, with or without jerking movements of the limbs. The word *convulsion* is used for the severe epileptic attack with unconsciousness and jerking. The word *attack* is used throughout the book as above, qualified by other words which indicate whether the event is epileptic or not. (In America *spell* is used in a similar way to *attack*.) *Seizure* is often used elsewhere as a synonym of fit, but in this book it is used to indicate a convulsive fit. *Blackout, syncope* and *faint* are used for non-epileptic attacks, unless there is some special explanation. Doctors often use two other words to describe epilepsy: *symptomatic* epilepsy and *idiopathic* epilepsy. Epilepsy is called *symptomatic* when the cause of the fits is known; for example, a scar in the brain. Epilepsy is called *idiopathic* when all known causes have been excluded. Idiopathic does not describe any special disease. It simply indicates that no cause or explanation can be found, even after thorough investigation.

The difficulties of those who suffer from fits

It is important to appreciate the difficulties of a patient who suffers from fits. The attacks themselves have a disturbing effect on the patient's life and may produce an understandable feeling of insecurity. An extract from the autobiography of Margiad Evans, *A Ray of Darkness*, may help the reader to grasp some of the sufferer's inner feelings. Margiad Evans first sensed something was wrong when consciousness was lost momentarily while crossing a room.

I went on with whatever I was doing, guided by the consciousness left over rather than the consciousness of the moment.... The whole thing took almost as long for a normal
person to walk five paces, say.

Some time later she had her first convulsion.

It was about about eleven o'clock when I put down my pen,
feeling suddenly tired and saying to myself that I could do no
more that night, so I would make a cup of tea and go to bed.
I made the tea, looked up at the clock—a strange chance—
and saw that it was ten minutes past eleven. The next moment
I was still looking up at the clock and the hands stood at five
and twenty minutes past midnight. I had fallen through Time,
Continuity and Being.

On recovering consciousness, Margiad had no inkling of
what had happened. The first thing she noticed was that one of
her sleeves was slightly charred by an ember from the fire. She
wanted to go to bed, but realised, shuddering, that she did not
know where it was, finding she could remember every room she
had slept in except the present one. Then Margiad became conscious of the fact that her clothes were damp, and with this
she at last knew the truth: she had had an epileptic fit.

Attacks may be frequent or infrequent, in public during the
daytime or when the patient is on his own in the middle of the
night. Uncertainty about when the next fit is due presents a
particular problem. A man with a weak leg—perhaps as a result
of poliomyelitis—always has his disability; a person with
epilepsy does not. Sometimes he has it and sometimes not, and
it may easily take him unawares.

Another problem is the response of the onlooker to the attack.
He may recoil in horror or even make fun of the sufferer. Many
times an epileptic person, on recovering from a fit, finds himself
in hospital, his whole pattern of life disrupted. He is also obliged
to take tablets regularly and though this is not in itself serious,
if a tablet is omitted a fit may follow this seemingly harmless
oversight. Sometimes the tablets themselves have a dulling

effect, producing unsteadiness or causing an unpleasant swelling of the gums.

Fits bar the sufferer from many practical and interesting occupations. They may also bar sufferers from work they feel strongly called to, such as nursing or the ministry. The person with epilepsy may not be allowed to drive a car and sometimes even riding a bicycle is forbidden by the doctor.

Leisure activities are therefore restricted as well as choice of work. Obviously the man subject to fits cannot go rock-climbing and sometimes it can be unwise even to swim. There are other troubles too: in certain parts of the world epileptics are forbidden to marry. In these and other places the epileptic is treated as if he were mad or some kind of a criminal. In spite of all these problems a great many people with epilepsy succeed in living almost normal lives.

Many people, apart from the family of the epileptic, are concerned with helping those in need. The general practitioner who has a number of epileptic patients on his list will prescribe treatment for them, and arrange for investigation in hospital if required. The teacher who has an epileptic child in her school will make arrangements for the best possible education. The social worker and the officers in the Labour Exchange may be involved in sorting out the special problems of family relationships and employment. The pharmacist feels challenged to discover new medications to control the fits. Even the geneticist may be called upon to explain the chances of a would-be parent's epilepsy being passed on to the child.

In fact anyone can be involved at any time, and to those who witness a fit, wherever it happens—the classroom, the street, the theatre or anywhere else—it means a cry for help. The onlooker usually has little idea of what is happening or what he can do for the best. It is one of the aims of this book to give him a better understanding of the condition and more sympathy for those suffering from epilepsy.

CHAPTER TWO

What causes fits?

WE HAVE no complete answer to the question: What is the cause of epilepsy? But in order to help us towards an answer the development, structure and working of the normal brain must be understood.

The development and structure of the brain

The brain results from the complex development process of the embryo within the mother's womb. A special tissue forms in the minute embryo from which most of the nervous system, including the brain, is derived. The stages of this development follow almost the same pattern in man as in much lower creatures. The primitive nervous tissue develops a swelling at one end, later to become the "head end", and on this swelling five distinct bulges appear. These continue to enlarge and modify, until the main areas of the brain are formed. The process has been completed by the end of the third month of pregnancy, when the primitive brain weighs less than a quarter of an ounce. As the embryo increases in size so does the brain, and at birth it already weighs eighteen ounces. The surface of the uppermost and largest part of the brain, the cerebrum, has a complex folded structure. It is divided into the left and right cerebral hemispheres.

What causes fits?

Deep in the cerebral hemispheres are masses of nervous tissue called the basal ganglia and thalamus. Below is the brain stem, which joins the hemispheres to the spinal cord. Each cerebral hemisphere is sub-divided into four lobes: the frontal, parietal, temporal and occipital lobes, which have their own special functions (figures 1 and 2).

The brain substance is composed of 10,000 million nerve

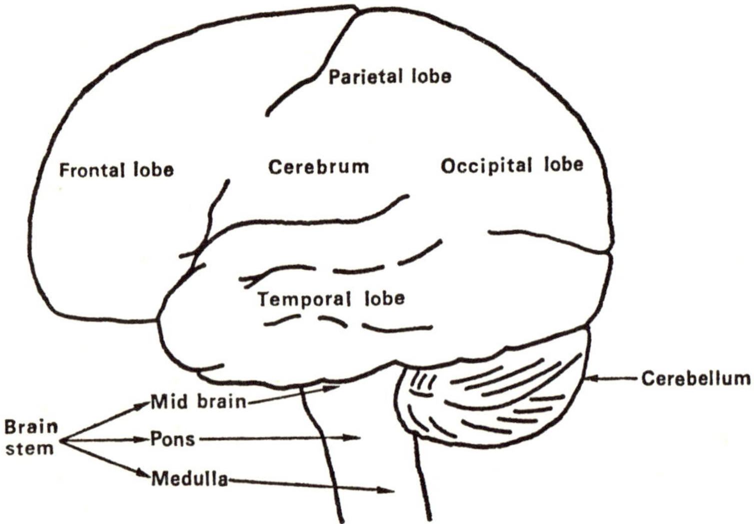

FIG. 1. The brain viewed from the side to show the main parts.

cells or neurones (figure 3). These consist of a cell body and a long fibre called an axon. These neurones are grouped so that their cell bodies lie either in the expanse of grey matter on the surface of the brain which is called the cortex, or in the smaller areas of grey matter deep inside the brain. The nerve fibres or axons which run from the cell bodies are grouped together into what is known as the "white matter". These fibres connect the cerebral hemispheres to other structures in the brain and the spinal cord. There are other cells in the brain which are distinct from the neurones. These are the neuroglia and their function is to support and nourish the nerve cells.

The whole brain is clothed in three covering layers called meninges. Between two of these layers is a space which contains the cerebro-spinal fluid. This forms in the hollow cavities inside the brain substance called ventricles (figure 4).

The brain is supplied with blood from the heart. It flows

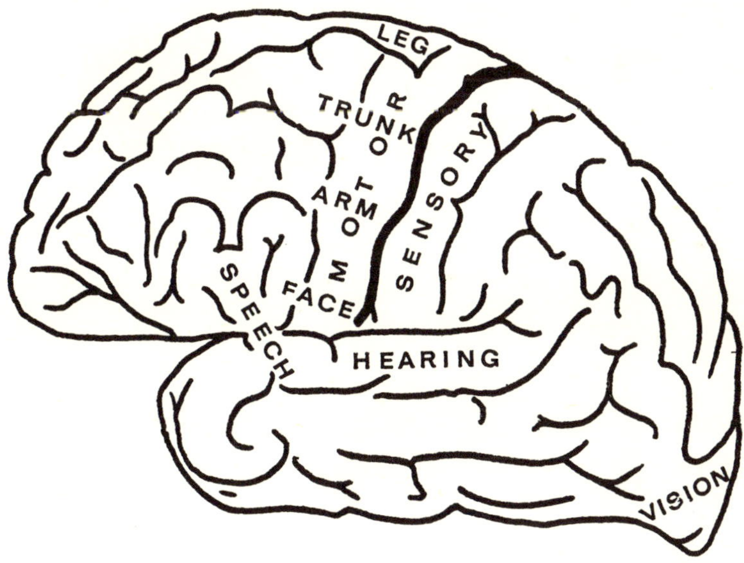

FIG. 2. The functional areas of the brain. The motor area is responsible for initiating movements.

through four large blood vessels which course up the neck, two at the front and two at the back. The blood vessels enter the skull and split into branches that fan out to supply different areas of the brain. They also form a complex network at the base of the brain so that if one of the blood vessels is damaged or blocked by disease, then blood can still reach that part of the brain supplied by the diseased vessel through other channels. Unfortunately, with age, this system of links between arteries becomes clogged and less efficient, and blockage of a vessel may then have serious effects.

The spinal cord, like the brain, consists of a mass of nerve cells arranged into grey and white matter. The spinal cord runs down from the brain in the middle of a tube formed by the vertebrae, and these bones together form the backbone. The

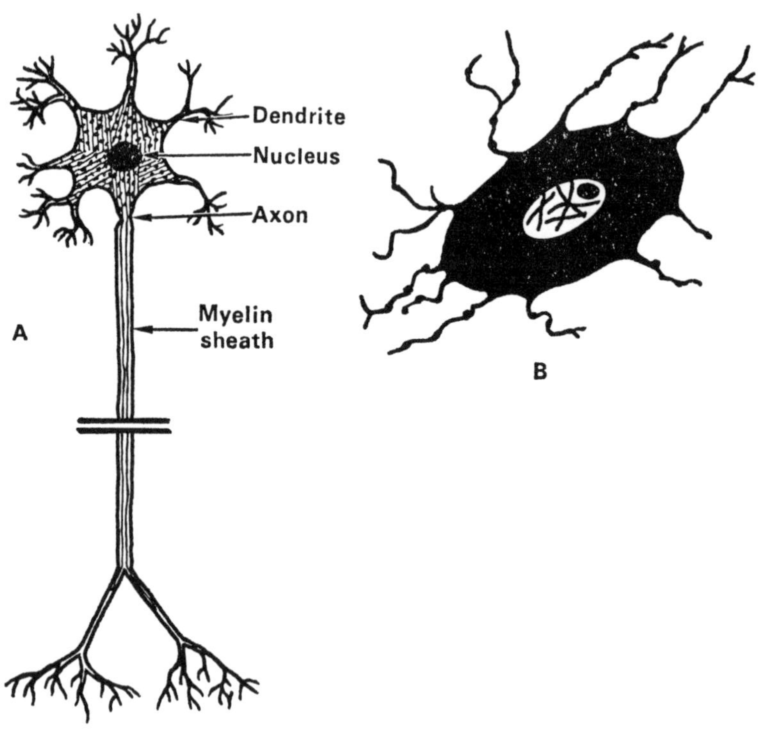

FIG. 3. Cells found in the brain and other parts of the nervous system.
A. A neurone.   B. A neuroglial cell.

coverings of the spinal cord lie within this tube or canal and, like those of the brain, are called meninges. They form a protective sheet for the delicate spinal cord. The fluid which is formed in the ventricles passes out on to the surface of the brain and then flows over the surface off the spinal cord within the meninges (figure 5). A specimen of fluid can be obtained by inserting a needle between the vertebrae into the spinal canal. Examination of the cerebro-spinal fluid is often very helpful in the diagnosis of diseases of the brain and spinal cord.

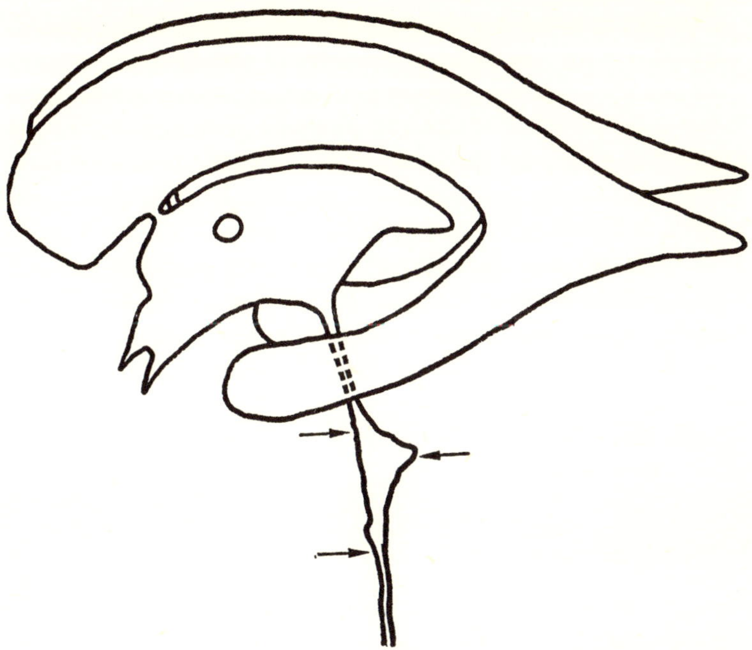

FIG. 4. An outline of the cavities called ventricles within the brain substance. Arrows indicate pores through which the cerebro-spinal fluid escapes to the surface of the brain.

The "life process" or metabolism of the brain

The cerebro-spinal fluid in conjunction with the meninges and the bony case of the skull form a protective covering for the brain. However, the brain also has a complex system of chemical protection, and it is here also that the cerebro-spinal fluid plays a part. When substances are injected into the bloodstream they quickly reach the tissues of the body. However, here the brain is an exception, for it is guarded by the "blood brain barrier" which prevents many substances in the blood from reaching the brain tissue. This barrier is formed by special neuroglial cells around the blood capillaries which feed the brain. These glial cells act as a selective—not a complete—food barrier, certain food substances, glucose in particular, being allowed to pass.

What causes fits?

The brain has a highly specialised and demanding system whereby energy for nervous processes is obtained. Two main materials are required, glucose and oxygen, which are brought to the brain by the bloodstream. As much as one-quarter of the total oxygen used by the body is employed by the brain even though that organ comprises only one-fiftieth of the total body weight. Because of its large requirements the brain is more sensitive to shortage than any other tissue. Of particular interest for our present purpose is the fact that during an epileptic fit the oxygen consumption of the brain may be increased by as much as 50 per cent. We can understand, therefore, that if a person suffers a series of fits in rapid succession a dangerous situation of oxygen starvation may arise in the brain, sometimes with extremely serious consequences.

Function of the nervous system

Though the nervous system is extremely complicated, its action depends upon very simple basic units which are linked together to produce complex responses. These simple action units are called reflexes and require only two or three neurones to form a reflex arc. One example of such a reflex action is when, for instance, a cook touches a hot stove and quickly withdraws her finger even before she has felt any pain: the reflex arc has brought about a reflex action. A nervous impulse has travelled from the cook's finger to the spinal cord interconnected with another nerve cell which has conveyed information to a muscle which then contracts. Another reflex arc is brought into action when the doctor tests the "knee jerk" (figure 5.)

However, more complicated movements are not dependent on reflex arcs alone, but require the intervention of the brain. In the frontal lobe of the cerebral hemisphere are located groups of nerve cells which form the frontal area. One collection of the cells in that area is responsible for initiating movements of the hand, another for initiating movements of the feet, and so on (figure 2). There are yet other areas—located in the parietal lobe of the cerebral hemisphere—which are responsible for receiving and interpreting sensations from the arms and the legs. Special sensations are not interpreted in the parietal lobe, but in their own special areas, in the case of vision in the occipital lobe, and for hearing in the temporal lobe.

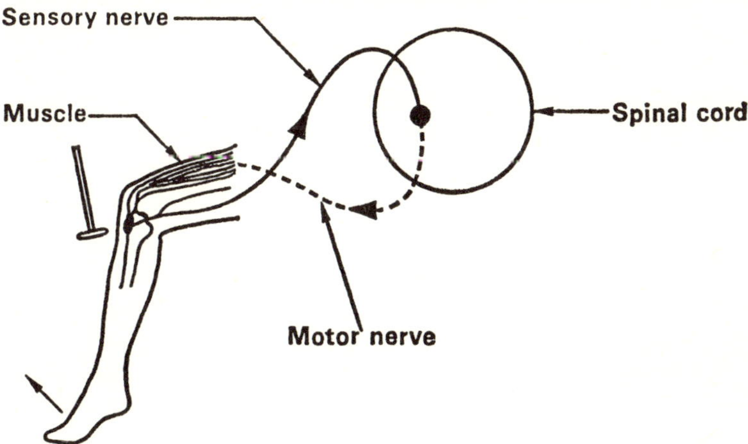

FIG. 5. An example of a reflex arc. The doctor taps the tendon with a small hammer, an impulse travels to the spinal cord and from there another impulse travels to the muscle, which contracts to produce the well-known knee-jerk.

Small electrical currents

All nervous activity is brought about by the passage of small electrical currents generated in the nerve cells, each of which has at least one branch or axon, which in turn has many smaller branches at the end. The cell bodies too have other branches and all these together act like electrical wires, joining one cell to many others. In this way groups of neurones can form circuits each with a different function.

The small electrical currents generated by brain cells can be recorded by placing electrodes, usually pads or discs, on the scalp. These electrical discharges are usually only a few millionths of a volt, but after amplification it is possible to record them with a pen writing on a continuous paper roll. This is known as an electro-encephalogram (EEG).

What causes fits?

Larger electrical discharges

Soon after this method was devised it was observed that patients with epilepsy had unusual electrical discharges not only during fits but in periods between them as well. Compared to normal discharges, those in epileptic people were of a much greater voltage, and the rate of the waves and their form were quite distinct. It was also observed that in a fit both the proper functioning and the electrical activity of the brain were disturbed. Sometimes these discharges could be seen to start in one area of the brain—say the zone responsible for hand movement—soon spreading to involve the rest of the arm and occasionally the whole body. Thus it can be concluded that a fit is a kind of miniature electrical storm in the brain which after reaching its peak dies away in a few seconds or minutes.

So it seems that those with epilepsy have brain cells which are more likely to have disordered electrical functions, and it is this which leads to seizures. However, a fit may be induced in a person not normally liable to them if a suitable provocative stimulus is used. The strong electrical current applied to the temples of patients with a depressive illness in the course of "shock treatment" is such a stimulus. This results in a major fit, but the violent muscular movements are controlled by a special paralysing drug. Potentially, it seems, everyone is an epileptic sufferer. Further, since there are electrical currents produced in the brain, it can be posited that the fact that some people are epileptic and others not is connected with some mechanism which damps down electrical activity and prevents its spread.

Consider the analogy of the heath fire: a match dropped in damp heather will quickly burn out, though after a long sunny day the same match will cause a serious fire. And just as it is the moisture in the undergrowth which prevents the spread of fire, so in the brain we believe there is a "damping mechanism" which controls the spread of electrical impulses. So far this mechanism has not been fully explained. A substance in the brain called gamma amino-butyric acid was once thought to have just this suppressing effect, but unfortunately it is not as straightforward as this and further research is needed on the subject.

Susceptibility to fits

One thing is certain: some people are more liable to fits than others. It has been suggested that the reason for this is that, in the former group, the brain cells are less able to suppress electrical discharges. It is possible that the defect in the cells is inherited, a view supported by the fact that the relatives of people with epilepsy often have an unusual pattern of brain activity (as recorded on the EEG) not unlike the epileptic's— even though they themselves are not subject to fits. It is observations like these which remind us of the complexity of epilepsy.

Some aspects of the mechanism whereby electrical discharges spread have been described and these general principles apply to any type of epilepsy. However, we must now examine the origin of the electrical discharges themselves. In some instances a definite cause can be found, while in others this is not yet possible.

Fits of known cause (symptomatic epilepsy)

Epilepsy is called symptomatic (see table 1) when both the cause of fits and the origin of the electrical discharges are understood. There are two kinds. In the first there is a definite brain disease, and it is the irritation of the surrounding cells which gives rise to the electrical discharges; these spread and a fit results. This source of electrical discharge is called a "focus", and may be caused by a head injury, perhaps at birth or as a result of a motor accident; in some instances an infection of the brain, such as meningitis, is responsible. In such cases, if the doctor succeeds in locating the focus it may then be possible in rare cases to cure the patient by surgery.

In the second variety of symptomatic epilepsy the disease process is not located in the brain but elsewhere in the body. A deficiency of oxygen because of some disease of the heart or lungs quickly disturbs the flow of oxygen to the brain and fits may sometimes occur.

Table 1. Types of symptomatic epilepsy

A. Disease of the brain

Tumours (cancerous or non-cancerous)
Head injury, at birth or later
Disease of blood vessels of the brain (cerebral arterio-sclerosis)
Inflammation of the brain (encephalitis) or its coverings (meningitis)
Rare disease present at birth (congenital), e.g. phenylke-tonuria, Sturge-Weber Syndrome.

B. Disease of the body affecting the brain

Heart disease
Febrile convulsions of childhood
Kidney disease
Hypoglycaemia (lowered blood sugar)
Various poisons, e.g. alcoholic beverages, lead, ergot

The constituents of the blood other than oxygen are upset in kidney disease, for example. The kidney is responsible for filtering off the waste products from the chemical processes of the body. When these organs fail the whole body, including the brain, is poisoned and again fits may occur.

Fits of unknown cause (idiopathic epilepsy)

Epilepsy is called idiopathic when no definite abnormality of the brain or disorder of the bodily system can be found and the site of origin of the fits in this condition cannot be determined.

If we know the age when a patient first began to have fits, this may help us to establish their cause. Most fits begin in the first twenty years of life. In fact, by that age, 80–90 per cent of all patients with epilepsy have begun their attacks, though fits may occur at any age, even into the nineties. If fits occur after the age of twenty there is a somewhat greater chance that a cause such as a scar may be discovered—symptomatic epilepsy. The reverse is also true: fits occurring before the age of twenty are less likely to be caused by a disease in the brain— the probability here is that one is dealing with idiopathic epilepsy. However, when attacks begin in the first year of life, there is a strong possibility that these are due to some congenital abnormality of the brain or to some injury at birth.

Poisons causing fits

A rare type of symptomatic epilepsy results when certain substances are taken orally or by injection. They are absorbed into the blood, carried to the brain and cause convulsions. Alcohol, for example, can cause fits in people who have never had them before; in fact, they may, though infrequently, follow a bout of drinking. The reason for this is not clear, but it is a fact that they often occur when the level of alcohol in the blood is falling. A possible factor is the occurrence in alcoholic drinks of substances which can harm the brain (see pp. 101–3). Yet another factor may be the relative starvation of many alcoholics when they are drinking heavily. They often take very little food and the consequent shortage of those substances which are required by the brain for proper functioning may increase the tendency to fits. In spite of these clues no definite explanation of fits following alcoholic bouts can be given.

Other substances too may cause fits by their effect on the brain, metallic lead being one such. Small children, with their tendency to lick paint or to chew on toy soldiers which contain lead, are particularly liable to fits. During the Middle Ages rye bread was frequently eaten, and in damp seasons this grain can become contaminated with the fungus *Claviceps purpurea*. As this fungus contains ergot, the bread in its turn contained this poison, and those who ate it developed burning pains in their hands and feet, probably because ergot causes contraction of the blood vessels. Another symptom of ergot poisoning was

What causes fits?

violent convulsions, presumably because blood vessels in the brain also contracted and restricted the flow of oxygen to the brain cells. It was particularly during times of famine (and even as late as the middle of the twentieth century, in France, when food was scarce) that ergot poisoning occurred.

In modern times there are some man-made chemicals which cause convulsions. Stimulants used by physicians to revive collapsed patients, if given in excessive amounts, may have this effect; nikethamide is one such substance. Pentylene tetrazol is the chemical name for another powerful substance, which though it can cause seizures has been employed to help in the diagnosis of epilepsy. In patients thought to have fits starting from a small area of the brain (i.e. focal fits) this substance is injected while the patient's EEG is recorded. If electrical discharges arise in the suspected part, the diagnosis of focal epilepsy is confirmed.

It is interesting to note that first camphor and then penthylene-tetrazol were used to produce fits in schizophrenic patients. This form of therapy—"shock treatment"—was used because it had been wrongly deduced that epilepsy and schizophrenia never occurred together in the same patient. We still employ shock treatment, but nowadays the shocks are given electrically, mainly for patients suffering from severe depression.

What can bring on fits?

In those prone to fits a number of circumstances may precipitate an attack. These precipitants are often indefinable; consequently research into the way in which they operate is difficult. However, emotional disturbances, lack of sleep, and certain stressful environments are often blamed for an increase in the frequency of attacks by the person who suffers from fits. Less nebulous factors are the changes associated with the menstrual cycle in women. As the cycle progresses fluid is retained in the body rather than passed out through the kidneys into the urine. This change is related to altering levels of hormones in the body. As a result some susceptible patients complain of fits in the few

20

days before the beginning of the menstrual flow, when the collection of fluid in the body is at its greatest. Then drugs which encourage the production of urine (diuretics) are useful for treatment in combination with the usual anti-epileptic tablets. During pregnancy there is also some retention of fluid, and as a result this too may be associated with increased frequency of fits in those susceptible. Another provocative stimulus is fever. Infants with a fever caused by tonsillitis or some ear infections may develop fits (see chapter VIII).

In order to function normally the nervous system requires (besides vitamins and oxygen) an adequate supply of glucose and calcium, which are carried, like the other substances in the blood, to the brain.

A diabetic patient gets up late, takes his usual dose of insulin but misses his breakfast. The level of glucose in his blood falls to a dangerously low level and the patient faints, the faint develops in severe cases into a fit, even in a diabetic not normally susceptible to them.

In a similar way if the blood calcium falls below the level required by the brain, a fit may occur. This disturbance of calcium in the body usually occurs with a complex hormonal upset. In neither the diabetic nor the patient with the calcium disturbance need there be anything abnormal in the brain, and an injection of the correct solution of either glucose or calcium would prevent the occurrence of further fits, until the same conditions occur again.

Effect of flashing lights

In numbers of instances complex stimuli may precipitate an attack in those who are susceptible. One at least was well known in ancient times. Apuleius implies that one common test before buying a slave was to make him observe the rotation of a potter's wheel and its flashing reflection. This is interesting, because in modern times badly adjusted televisions have been known to bring on a fit. The electro-encephalographer makes use of a similar technique (see chapter IV), using a bright regular flashing light to provoke epileptic discharges in EEG recording. Some small children who have minor epileptic fits and are sensitive to flashing lights have formed the habit of bringing on an attack themselves by moving their hands (fingers spread wide apart) in front of their eyes when looking at the sun. Another form of stimulation that may in rare cases cause fits is reading. Yet others are musical sounds and loud and unexpected noises. But it is only rarely that these stimuli actually bring on an attack, even among people susceptible to epilepsy.

CHAPTER THREE

What sorts of fits are there?

FITS, THEN, are the result of sudden and abnormal electrical activity in the brain. Depending on where these electrical disturbances begin, where they spread, and how fast they spread, so the pattern of the fit is determined. Though it is still disputed how best to classify fits, an international classification has now been completed (see pp. 151–3).

The commonest type of fit is the convulsion, and it is the suddenness and violence of this type that impresses the layman. However, there are many other kinds less impressive to the observer but equally disturbing to the person who suffers from them. In fact many people with epilepsy never have a convulsion, while some have them only infrequently or just once in their lives. A particular epileptic patient may have one or many different types of attack, though it is usual for one patient to have only one kind.

The convulsion or "grand mal" attack

Doctors call an attack in which convulsions and complete unconsciousness occurs a *"grand mal"*, or major attack. It is the commonest fit in adolescence and adults, though it occurs in children too, and accounts for about 50 per cent of all fits.

Depending on whether the warning is long-lasting or brief, the name *prodrome* or *aura* is applied to it. A prodrome is a sensation lasting for several hours before an attack, a feeling, for example, of tension, depression or, less commonly, excitement or elation. Dostoevsky experienced this elation throughout the day preceding his epileptic seizures. As he describes it, through the character of Prince Myshkin in *The Idiot*: "all his emotions, all his doubts, all his anxiety calmed together to be changed in a sovereign serenity made up of lighted joy, harmony and hope; then his reason was raised up to the understanding of the final cause".

Much more common is the occurrence of a very brief warning or aura, which electrical studies of the brain show to be the beginning of the attack itself. There are a great variety of auras, for example, a strange smell, like burning sulphur, or a tingling in the hands, similar to the common sensation of pins and needles. Though it can be frightening, the aura can also be useful, for it gives the sufferer time to lie down, so that at least he will not fall and hurt himself when the attack begins. There may even be time for him to remove his false teeth. The aura leads immediately into the "tonic" stage of the fit, so called because there is rigid contraction of the muscles of the chest and of the rest of the body. Air is then forced through the larynx or voice box and the cry which is automatically produced indicates only that the attack has actually begun, not that the sufferer is in pain. For about half a minute the arms and legs remain stiff and the chest is motionless. As breathing has ceased no oxygen enters the lungs and the face later becomes blue-grey in colour. The heart, however, continues to beat unaltered.

Suddenly the tonic phase leads into the jerking or "clonic" stage of the fit. The jaws jerk and the tongue is often bitten. A blood-stained foam collects on the lips and in the corners of the mouth. At this stage too, the patient often passes urine or exceptionally, soils himself, because of the violent contractions. Marked jerking of the arms, legs and trunk muscles also occurs, and the head sometimes bangs on the floor, also as a result of the muscular contractions. The movements die away, leaving the body limp. The breathing, which may have stopped, momentarily deepens, and the person lies apparently lifeless.

Following such a convulsion the sufferer usually passes imperceptibly from unconsciousness into a deep sleep which can last from a few minutes to several hours. If this sleep does not follow, the person may, on recovery, complain of a headache or be confused for a minute or two. It will be obvious that, as he was completely unconscious during the fit, he will have absolutely no memory of it.

This description of a convulsion indicates that an epileptic attack can be divided into three parts: first the warning, secondly the actual fit itself, thirdly the recovery. In the case of the convulsion, the fit itself has a tonic, followed by a clonic stage.

The "petit mal"

The "*petit mal*" attack, which is the simplest and briefest kind of fit, usually occurs without warning and has no recovery stage. The bystander, in fact, may hardly notice anything. This type of attack, which is merely a brief lapse of full consciousness, is commonest in childhood. If the attack is sufficiently brief, the person is often unaware that anything has happened to him.

Such an attack is quite different from the sudden, overwhelming convulsion, and can pass by completely unnoticed. The patient may falter in his conversation—but then many people without epilepsy do this, and the momentary, vacant pause, sometimes accompanied by a fluttering of the eyelids, can easily be shrugged off. These small attacks are most frequent in the morning on rising, though there may be many hundreds throughout the course of the day. By contrast, it is uncommon for more than one convulsive attack to occur in one day.

In some patients the slight jerking of the arms and legs, often a part of the *petit mal* attack, may be very pronounced. These purposeless movements, known as myoclonic jerks, may then affect not only the arms and legs but the trunk muscles as well.

What sorts of fits are there?

The affected person may then lose his balance and be thrown to the floor. There is no warning at all of such an attack and injuries are common. Again, these spasms are usually seen in young children and it is likely that a child subject to such fits will suffer from the convulsive ones as well.

Perhaps it is as well to note here that many people suffer from similar jerking movements of the legs as they fall asleep. These jerks are a common occurrence and have nothing to do with epilepsy.

Jacksonian attacks

In both convulsive seizures and *petit mal* attacks the patient's awareness of his surroundings is altered. In the first he becomes unconscious, and in the second, although he rarely blacks out altogether, he never knows quite where he is or what is happening. In another form of attack the patient can give an accurate account of the experience because he remains completely alert throughout. These attacks sometimes begin with a tingling in the hand or the involuntary movement of a thumb. The sensation or movement spreads from the extremity along all the affected limbs. This is particularly interesting, because the electrical discharge in the brain that accompanies such an attack spreads likewise from the foot or hand area of the frontal lobe to the shoulder or hip area. Sometimes a Jacksonian attack heralds a convulsive fit, but more often it dies away after a few seconds or minutes. Usually the limb affected may feel weak for a few hours or even a few days afterwards. The Jacksonian fit is the most infrequent of all.

The psychomotor fit

A psychomotor fit, like the Jacksonian fit, begins in one small part of the brain. It is the commonest type of attack after the convulsion, and accounts for as many as 35–40 per cent of all fits. The part of the brain involved varies from patient to patient, but generally the focus is in the temporal lobe of the brain so called because it lies behind the temple, mainly on the under-surface of the brain. As in Jacksonian fits the electrical discharge in the brain during the psychomotor fit may spread slowly and without causing a convulsion.

The most frequent sensation at the beginning of a temporal lobe attack is a curious feeling in the pit of the stomach which rises towards the throat. The patient may sometimes notice an unpleasant indescribable odour, or hear familiar voices or a noise like the ringing of bells.

As, it seems, some aspects of memory are stored in parts of the temporal lobe, complex events, often vivid scenes from child-hood, may suddenly be relived in the mind without the person making any effort to recall them.

Two other disturbances of memory may occur. The first is an intense feeling of familiarity despite the fact that the patient's environment at the time is entirely new. The feeling of "I have been here before" is perhaps the best way to describe this sensation known as "*déjà vu*". (It may also occur in people without epilepsy who are fatigued or under emotional stress.) The second is a sensation of unfamiliarity even though the person is in a perfectly familiar place, e.g. in his own home, a feeling which the French call "*jamais vu*". Although psycho-motor attacks usually (but not always) occur in patients with temporal lobe epilepsy, these patients may have other types of attacks too, e.g. *grand mal*. However, because the occurrence of psychomotor attacks with temporal lobe epilepsy is so common, the two can for the most part be considered together.

Our description of the psychomotor attack has so far included only the feelings of the sufferer, not what the observer sees. During the attack the onlooker may find it difficult to be sure what has happened—even whether the person is having a fit or not—so great is the variety of phenomena seen: the person might stop what he is doing, stare vacantly and then begin some repetitive movement such as stroking his hair, clutching at the bedclothes, or rubbing his leg; he may turn his head or eyes to one side as though his attention has been attracted by a noise; sometimes he stretches out an arm to grasp an invisible object. The empty mouth may make chewing movements. Mumbled words are heard, short, repeated phrases such as "Where's the wife?" or "I'm not, I'm not".

During a psychomotor attack the patient is not unconscious but in a kind of dream. On recovering, he remembers little of what actually happened during the attack, sometimes nothing at all. Normal behaviour is resumed over a matter of minutes.

An attack like this is called an automatism because the person behaves like an automaton. It also occurs in patients after a major fit, and sometimes this alteration in the awareness of events may develop into what is known as a "fugue state". These states occur not only in epileptic patients, but also sometimes after head injury, in some forms of depression, and in other mental illnesses. In these states when consciousness is not clear, complex acts may occur, such as walking down the street, buying cigarettes, travelling considerable distances. The observer will find the patient looking almost normal, though he will probably be pushed firmly aside if he tries to intervene. These "fugues", though very rare, provoke great interest in legal circles, because it is theoretically possible that unlawful acts can be performed during them, and they may be used as a defence by a clever criminal (see chapter XIII).

Almost any fit, except the *petit mal* or Jacksonian varieties, ends with sleep, a headache or a few minutes of muddleheadedness. Work or play begins again almost at once, so much so that a person who has several attacks in the day may still be able to continue working efficiently.

Status epilepticus

Rarely, one convulsion may follow another, without consciousness being regained. This condition is called "status epilepticus". Because of the repeated fits the brain quickly becomes starved of both oxygen and glucose; this, coupled with an inability to take solid nourishment or liquids, is very serious, and the patient has to be admitted urgently to hospital for treatment.

More rarely *petit mal* attacks may occur one after the other, a condition called *"petit mal* status". This is not serious and can usually be treated by the doctor, without the patient needing to stay in hospital.

Other kinds of fits

There are still other types of focal fits. In one sort, as a result of an epileptic discharge in one cerebral hemisphere, the person's head and eyes turn automatically to the side. Sometimes an arm is raised at the shoulder, or the leg stretched out. In other attacks these rather simple movements may be replaced by complicated movements such as walking round and round in a small circle. Such epileptic manifestations are called "adversive fits".

Another kind of attack occurs only in very young children and it is produced by generalised brain disease. There is a sudden thrusting movement of the arms, while at the same time the body, and sometimes the head, jerks forward. This condition is called "infantile spasm" and is often associated with mental retardation (see chapter IX).

To summarise, fits may be major or minor. The major attack, which leads to complete loss of consciousness, is called a *grand mal*, or convulsion. The minor attack includes all other types of epileptic attack, such as the *petit mal*, psychomotor, Jacksonian or temporal lobe attack.

Another way of classifying fits is to think of them as either generalised or focal. The generalised attacks, *grand mal* and *petit mal*, involve the whole brain in varying degrees from the start. Focal or partial fits, to give them another name, start in one part of the brain, and the pattern of the attack depends on the site of the abnormal discharge. A Jacksonian attack often begins in the motor area of the brain responsible for movements of the body. The psychomotor fit usually starts in the temporal lobe concerned with hearing, smell and some aspects of memory.

The main kinds of fits and their classification have been given.

However, fits do not all fall neatly into categories and it may take years for even a doctor to realise that a person with some odd behaviour suffers, in fact, from epilepsy. Fits are usually sudden and different but they are not always so, and epileptic phenomena may therefore shade imperceptibly into normal behaviour.

CHAPTER FOUR

The diagnosis of fits

SINCE FITS, faints and falls are often inextricably intertwined, a patient having an attack which may be a fit requires a thorough investigation. This will include finding out whether the attack is epileptic and, if so, which type of epilepsy is present and whether or not the cause can be found.

A policeman investigating a road accident begins by questioning witnesses and continues by examination of the scene of the accident, while later laboratory investigations may be carried out. The doctor starts his diagnosis by obtaining information from the patient and his relatives.

What sort of attack?

First of all, a description of the fit is obtained from the patient. He is asked what led up to the fit, what he knew of it, and what happened afterwards. Was he in bed, at work, or in the street; hungry, tired, in an emotional state, or under the influence of alcohol? The whole complicated interrogation continues with questions about previous illnesses in childhood and since. Even details of birth are important, for head injuries at birth can be extremely relevant. Enquiries are also made to discover whether similar fits or other kinds of illness run in the family.

The diagnosis of fits

Next, an eyewitness account is sought, and the wife, parent or workmate is questioned. Gradually the setting of the attack, its nature and termination are brought together.

The examination begins

The first investigation over, the physician begins his physical examination of the patient. The nervous system is checked and hearing, vision and taste are examined. The power of the limbs, the reflexes and other functions are tested. Results may reveal the presence of a tumour in the brain, or the sequel of previous brain injury. Next, the examination moves on to other parts of the body, including the heart and lungs. A diseased heart, for instance, may beat slowly, resulting in the brain being starved of blood, a condition which may cause fits.

X-ray examinations

Further investigation of the brain by laboratory tests is obviously difficult. The brain is encased in its skull, and routine X-rays will rarely reveal changes in the brain itself. Special X-ray techniques may therefore be necessary. In order to outline the brain, air has to be inserted into the hollow spaces, or ventricles, inside the skull. This is usually done by performing a lumbar puncture. A needle is introduced in the lower back between the vertebral bones, and some of the fluid which bathes the spinal cord drained off. This fluid, as we have already mentioned (p. 12), also bathes the brain, and laboratory tests may give information valuable to the diagnosis. Immediately after the doctor has drawn off the fluid some air is injected, with the patient sitting upright. As the air is lighter than the fluid it rises, surrounds the brain and enters the ventricular cavities. Distortions caused by tumours or scars or other disease (see figure 6) are thus outlined and can be seen as shadows on the X-ray photographs which are then taken.

There is another way of tackling the investigation of the brain using X-rays. This time a substance is injected into a blood

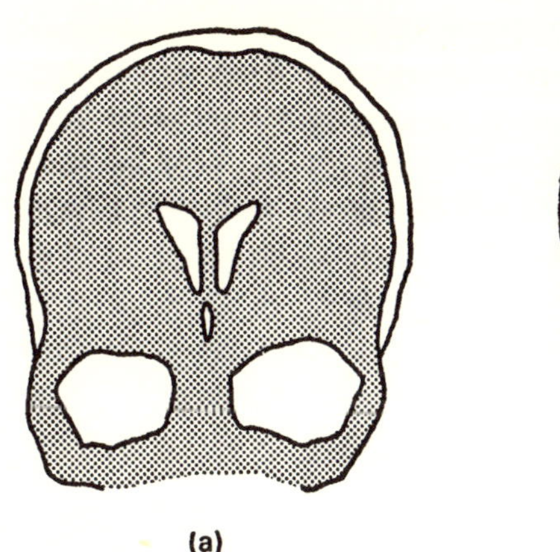
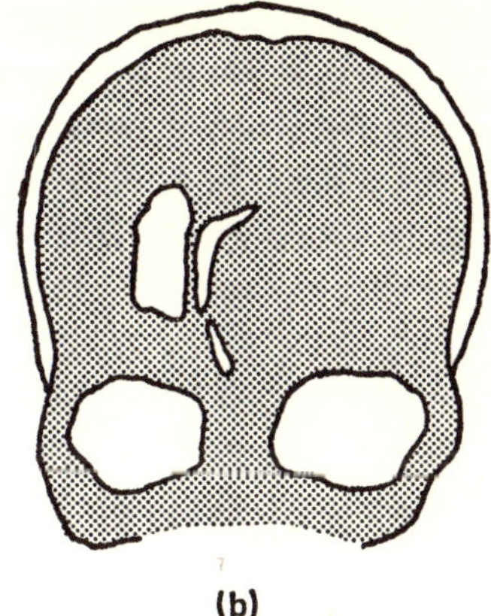

FIG. 6.

(a) The normal ventricles as seen on an X-ray photograph after injection of air.
(b) The effects of a cerebral tumour on the left side with distortion of the ventricular pattern.

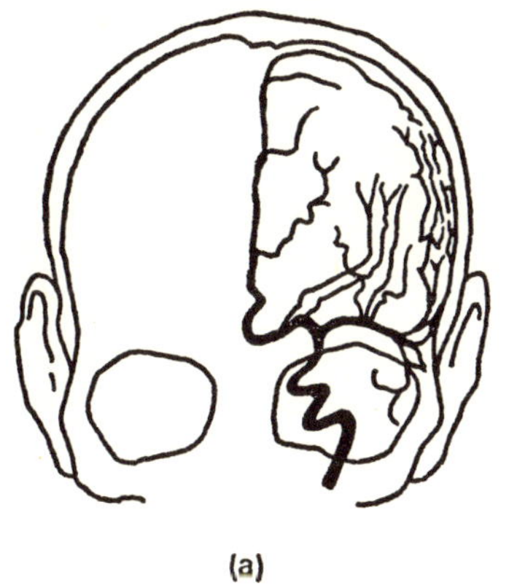
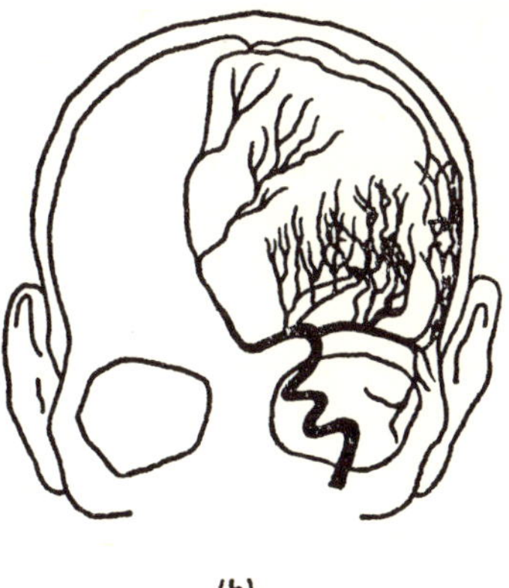

FIG. 7.

(a) The pattern obtained on an X-ray photograph when the blood vessels of the brain are outlined by a special substance.
(b) A tumour on the left side of the brain is demonstrated with the resulting distortion of the vessel pattern.

vessel in the neck. This substance is carried quickly to the blood vessels of the brain, making them stand out as shadows when the X-ray photograph is developed, and again a tumour or other brain disease will be shown up (figure 7). Not only do these X-ray investigations indicate whether brain disease is present or not, but they can often locate it exactly. Though these tests sound extremely unpleasant and require a few days in hospital, they are quite harmless.

The electro-encephalogram (EEG)

Perhaps the most important test on the patient suspected of epilepsy is the electro-encephalogram—the E E G. This method of recording the electrical activity of the brain has a long history.

As early as 1875 Caton showed that electrical activity in the brains of animals could be demonstrated; but because photography was in its infancy he was not able to produce permanent records. However, he was able to persuade the British Medical Association of the importance of his work, and they gave him a grant so that he would continue his research; but it was not until many years later, after much secret investigation, particularly on the brain rhythms of his son, that Hans Berger in 1929 published reports of the human E E G. Since that time the technique has been greatly improved and now many different patterns of brain activity have been documented. The actual recording machine is quite large and complicated and may be frightening to children, but in fact the test is harmless, since it is only the recording of electrical current that is carried out; no electrical discharge is passed from the equipment into the patient. The waves from the brain are amplified about 100,000 times and are then written out on a moving paper strip so that a permanent record is obtained. The results are similar to, but vastly more complicated than, the recording of electrical activity in the heart on an electro-cardiogram, because the waves from several areas of the brain are recorded simultaneously and vary from one another.

Usually no special preparation is required before an E E G is performed and it can be carried out without admission to hospital. Electrodes are attached to the scalp, either silver discs with glue, or pads soaked in salt water covering the ends of silver rods, held in place with a firm rubber net. The electrodes are then attached by wires to the E E G recording machine. About twenty electrodes in all are used so that activity from

Kind of Activity	*Form and Frequency*	*Remarks*
Alpha	8–14 cycles/sec.	Normal activity seen at back of the head.
Beta	above 14 cycles/sec.	Normal activity. Marked increase with anti-convulsant medicines.
Theta	4–7 cycles/sec.	Occurs in drowsiness and many diseases.
Delta	below 4 cycles/sec.	Occurs in deep sleep, also in many disorders including brain tumours.
Spikes		Occurs in patients with epilepsy.
Spike and Wave		Occurs mainly in children with 'petit mal' attacks.

Fig. 8. Samples of different kinds of normal and abnormal E E G activity. Each tracing represents about 1 second of recording.

all over the brain can be sampled at once. The patient relaxes on a couch while the recording is carried out, and the whole procedure takes from half an hour to an hour.

Normal "brain waves"

When Berger first described the E E G, because of the simplicity of the apparatus at his disposal he was only able to record from one area of the brain. Later, with better apparatus, it was

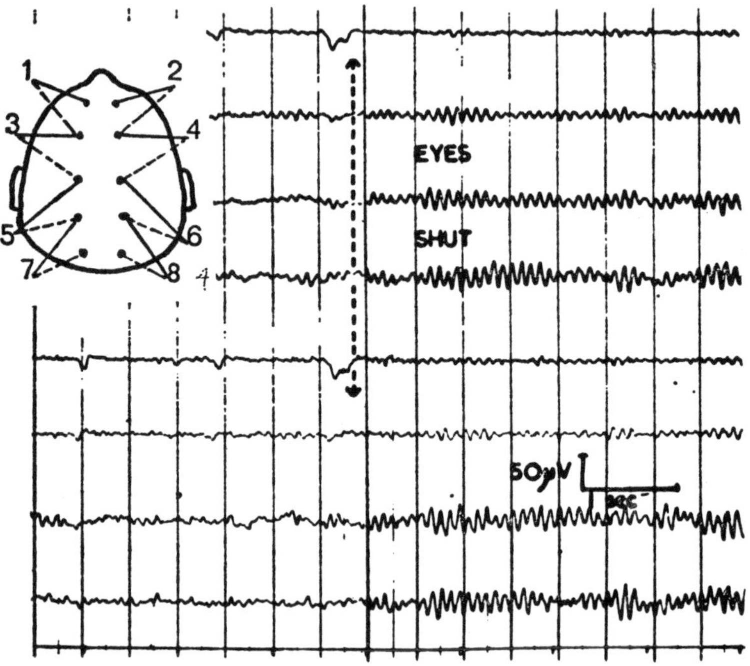

FIG. 9. A normal adult E E G. The alpha rhythm at 10 cycles per second is seen when the eyes are closed. It is "blocked" by eye opening, as shown in the first part of the recording.

observed that activity from different parts of the brain was different in form. From the back of the head, fairly large regular waves at the rate of about ten per second were seen, while from the front and middle of the head smaller waves at about twice that frequency occurred. The ten cycles per second waves were called the alpha rhythm, and the faster waves the beta rhythm (figure 8). Both these rhythms appear in the EEGs of most adults. The alpha rhythm is particularly interesting because when the eyes are opened it disappears almost completely. It may disappear (figure 9) if the eyes remain closed and the person is asked to make simple arithmetical calculations. This does not mean that the EEG measures intelligence or personality.

In children, the EEG pattern differs from that seen in adults. In the first month of life there is very little activity seen at all

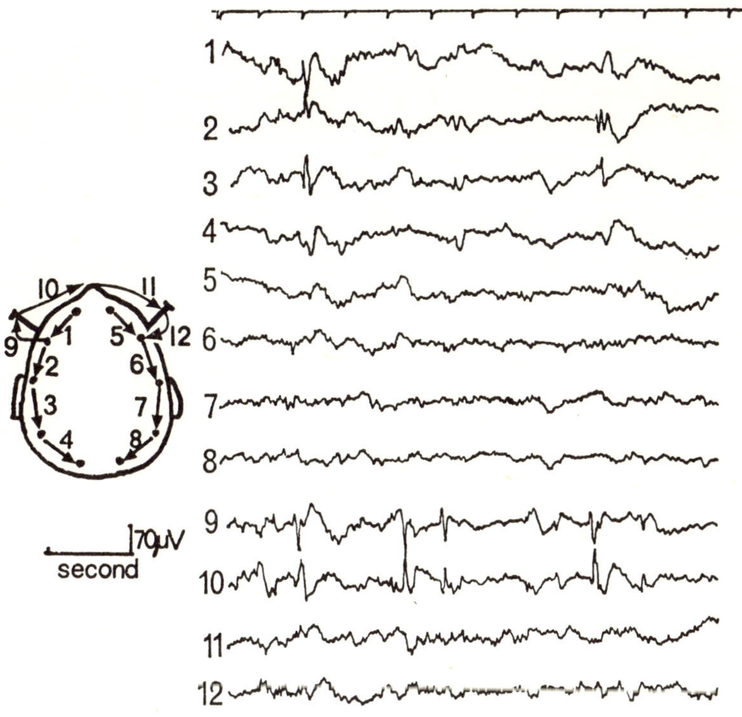

FIG. 10. The EEG of a man with temporal lobe epilepsy. He is aged twenty-three years and experienced attacks of intense fear sometimes followed by unconsciousness. The EEG shows frequent spike activity particularly coming from the left temporal lobe as shown in the channels numbered 1–3, 9 and 10.

and none appears at the back of the head, where the normal adult alpha rhythm occurs. As the infant gets older traces of alpha-like activity are seen in the centre of the head, and with increasing age the pattern gets more and more like the adult's. The reason for these changes of EEG are not known. However, it is thought that they are related to maturation of the brain cells, which continues after birth. By about fifteen years the child's EEG is indistinguishable from that of an adult. There is no clear relationship between the development of the EEG and a child's bone structure or mental ability.

Epileptic brain waves

People with epilepsy have both alpha and beta rhythms, but in addition they show other phenomena which are not like those regular waves described. They are large, sudden and irregular. In the case of temporal lobe epilepsy (figure 10), frequent sharp waves occur, while patients with *petit mal* attacks (figure 11) have discharges called "spike" and "wave" in their EEGs. Sometimes in addition epileptic patients show waves at a

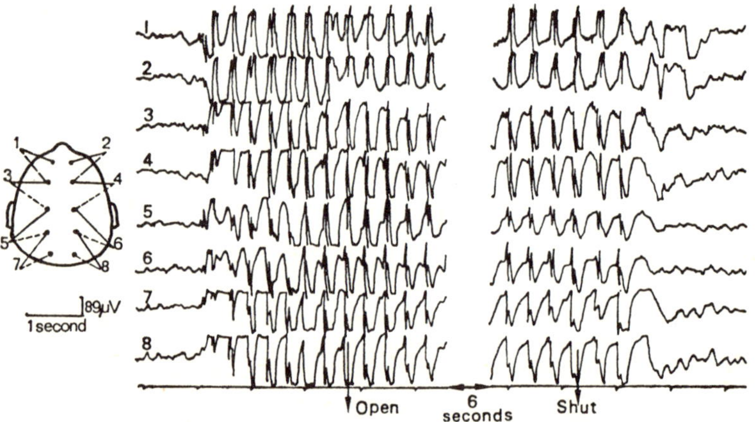

Fig. 11. The EEG of a boy during a *petit mal* attack. He stares, looks vacant and for a few seconds his arms and legs twitch. During the recording he was asked to shut his eyes but did not respond for several seconds.

much slower frequency than the alpha rhythm, and these are
called either theta or delta waves, depending on whether they
are slow or very slow. These occur not only in epilepsy but also
in many other diseases, including some types of brain tumour
(figure 12).

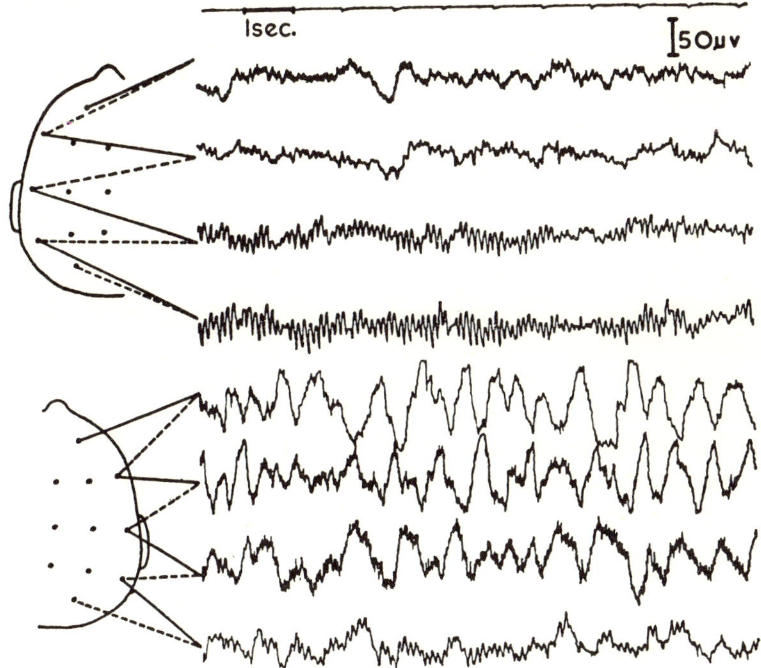

FIG. 12. The effect of cerebral tumour on the EEG. The lower four
tracings are from the right side of the brain and show a widespread disturbance with the occurrence of delta activity. About 20 per cent of all
patients with cerebral tumours suffer from epilepsy as well as showing this
abnormal pattern.

Flickering lights

At some stage in the EEG examination, in order to bring out
epileptic activity the patient is asked to breathe deeply and
rapidly in and out for a period of about three minutes. At
another stage during the examination the recordist puts a
special lamp in front of the patient about a foot away from his

face. This electronic device, known as a stroboscope, produces a series of rapid, very short, extremely brilliant flashes of light. The frequency of the flash is determined by the turn of a knob. It has been shown that each bright flash produces a corresponding wave in the brain of almost anyone. This response is recorded from the back of the head which lies over the occipital lobe, the receiving and sorting area for visual information. Information enters through the eye and reaches this remote part of the brain after a series of complicated connections. In some epileptic patients an abnormal pattern arises in response to the flashing light. The normal response remains localised to the brain, but the epileptic response seen in some patients spreads and takes the form of "spike and wave", which we know as a characteristic epileptic discharge. Just occasionally this type of response is seen in patients without epilepsy, which makes diagnosis rather more difficult.

This flicker response, which indicates sensitivity to light in some epileptic patients, is more than of just academic interest. It helps us to understand what happens when a child has a fit in front of a badly adjusted television set which is flashing, or when the pilot of a propellor-driven plane "blacks out" in a convulsive seizure because the sunlight is broken up by the propellor blade, or when a motorist has a fit while driving along an avenue of trees with the sun shining behind them.

Sometimes a patient with epilepsy may have a normal EEG. Then other methods of investigation are required. A recording after a sleeping tablet is carried out since sleep may provoke epileptic discharges. If this is unsuccessful special types of electrode are used to record from areas of the brain not reached by the standard scalp electrodes.

Conversely, some people who do not have fits may show patterns in their EEG not dissimilar to those occurring in epileptic patients. These patterns may occur in as many as 5–10 per cent of normal subjects. They are even more frequent in the relatives of epileptic patients who do not themselves have fits. However, in spite of these limitations, the EEG is valuable because specific changes can be recorded in patients who have brain tumours or other diseases of the brain which may be the cause of symptomatic epilepsy.

The EEG is a harmless test which will usually indicate whether the attack was a faint or a fit and, further, may suggest the nature of the abnormality causing it.

Other tests

Other tests have been devised more recently to investigate the brain, particularly tumours. One such test makes use of high frequency waves as used in radar. The coverings of the brain and the brain itself reflect these waves and any distortion can be demonstrated. Another test makes use of radioactive isotopes. Following injection into the blood, these substances are absorbed by growing tumour tissue, for example in the brain. Radioactive isotopes emit rays which can be picked up by a special counter, so that a tumour, if present, can be detected and its position plotted. The results of both these valuable techniques have been examined in various specialist hospitals and they are now generally available.

One or two fits

The occurrence of one or two fits puts the doctor very much on his guard. It is often very difficult to discover the cause without putting the patient through a whole series of investigations. If the patient is an infant suffering from a cold or tonsillitis, then probably little enquiry is needed, though this is a matter of opinion. Some doctors will arrange for the EEG in these circumstances and begin treatment with anti-convulsant drugs. Here, as well as in other areas of the care of the epileptic patient, knowledge is limited and doctors go by their experience rather than by strict rules.

For the older patient who has one or two fits after the age of twenty-five it is generally considered that a great deal of investigation should be undertaken, for after this age epilepsy appearing for the first time might be found to be symptomatic. A fit may be the first sign of a brain tumour or some other, rarer disease. A single convulsion without an aura or warning is usually less significant in this connection than a "focal" fit. Such a fit, beginning in one defined area of the brain, almost certainly indicates disease there. The careful collection of exact information about the type of fit, the circumstances and the after-effects are, as usual, very important. The doctor must find out too whether similar attacks have ever occurred in the family. In the case of focal fits it may be necessary to undertake more extensive investigations but certainly an EEG will be performed. This type of attack may sometimes be treatable by surgery or other means.

In summary, the diagnosis of epilepsy depends on a careful collection of evidence from the patient and his relatives, by examination and special tests. As a result it should be possible to institute the appropriate treatment and in many instances forecast the outcome (prognosis).

CHAPTER FIVE

Faints and falls

MANY DISORDERS appear under the guise of epilepsy. Sometimes it is easy to sort out the fits from the faints and falls, but sometimes it is almost impossible. Let us now examine some of these attacks which are not fits.

Fainting attacks

Faints are sometimes confused with fits, not because they are particularly similar but because faints are more acceptable to the patient and his family. In fact, a fainting attack (syncope) is usually quite easily distinguished from an epileptic attack.

The patient is often a child who may have been standing for a long time waiting for a meal. The first sensations of a faint are a feeling of light-headedness, of sickness, and weakness of the legs. The patient becomes pale and sweat stands out on his brow. He sways, yawns, and then sinks slowly and limply to the floor. He loses consciousness, but only briefly, and his breathing, often shallow, is interspersed with sighing. When after a minute or two he opens his eyes he may complain of headache or nausea. He may even vomit. In almost all cases there is little or no muscular movement of the arms or legs, no tongue biting or loss of control of the urine. He may sleep off his faint but commonly, after a short period of lying flat, the unpleasant sensations pass. This is normally quite unlike the recovery stage of a patient who has just had a fit. Such a patient usually sleeps for half an hour or even longer.

The faint is usually caused by blood pooling in the legs because of prolonged standing. Remember our guardsman? As blood does not return promptly to the heart, enough of it is not pumped out to maintain the oxygen supply to the brain.

Attacks caused by pressure on the carotid sinus

Another type of attack may be brought on by the stimulation of a small nerve centre in the wall of one of the arteries of the neck. It is called the carotid sinus and is responsible for maintaining blood pressure. Nervous impulses travel between this centre and blood vessels in other parts of the body. If the blood pressure rises, the centre transmits a signal to the vessels so that they enlarge slightly causing pressure to fall in them, and vice versa.

In some people, however, this centre is particularly sensitive to stimulation by external pressure. Even a tight collar is enough to start an attack when the person turns his head. When this happens messages pass to the blood vessels, which expand very rapidly. The pressure in the blood vessels suddenly falls, the brain is starved of blood and fainting occurs. When trying to reach an accurate diagnosis of attacks which may be faints or fits, a physician will often press on the patient's neck to try and produce an attack. In both faints, whether due to carotid sinus stimulation or not, the EEG is normal except during the attack itself, but then the pattern is quite different from that seen during an epileptic fit.

Attacks resulting from a slow heart beat

The heart usually beats 70–80 times a minute, though in some athletes at the peak of their training the rate may fall to as low as 40–50 beats. However, when there is disease of the heart the system which regulates the beating may be upset. As a result the rate may suddenly fall. Then an adequate supply of blood does not reach the brain and a special type of faint results, known as a Stokes-Adams attack after the two doctors who first described it. The physician must administer stimulating injections of nikethamide or adrenaline to the heart, when the beat quickly returns to its normal rate. If the heart fails to speed up, the blood supply and therefore oxygen supply to the brain will become seriously depleted and a true epileptic fit may follow. Nowadays an artificial pacemaker can be embedded below the skin near the heart to keep its beat normal in patients who suffer from Stokes-Adams attacks.

Breath-holding attacks

Infants have another attack which may be confused with fits—breath-holding spells. A frustrated infant, usually between one and two years old, holds his breath after a spell of crying. In a few seconds he turns blue and falls to the floor. He may lie there limp and motionless, his lips purplish in appearance. Rarely, he jerks and after a few frightening minutes he recovers. These breath-holding spells are usually quite easily distinguishable from fits, which occur without provocation and in which there are definite jerking movements. The EEG in the child with epilepsy is usually abnormal, while the infant with breath-holding spells does not have any definite changes in the EEG between attacks. The child usually grows out of breath-holding spells, and there are no after-effects.

In older children temper tantrums occur. These are not the result of epileptic discharges in the brain, and in this sense are like the so-called "brainstorm" or "fit of rage", seen in adults. They are usually associated with abnormalities of the personality rather than with epilepsy. Of course, a person who suffers from epilepsy may suffer from attacks of rage, but no more so than a person without fits.

Sleeping attacks

Narcolepsy is a rare disease which is not related to epilepsy but may be confused with it. A person with narcolepsy has an overwhelming and uncontrollable desire to sleep, and the sufferer may remain deeply asleep for long periods. For example, a housewife nods off as soon as her husband leaves for work after breakfast. He returns in the evening to find no meal prepared for him and his wife asleep in the chair. A small regular dose of a stimulant drug may, however, be sufficient to prevent these troublesome narcoleptic attacks and improve marital harmony! Another side of this rare complaint is the occurrence of cataplexy. Here, extreme weakness of the body occurs, precipitated by a strong emotion like laughter; for such a person a good joke can be a serious matter. This astonishing state of affairs can usually be corrected by the same type of stimulant drug as for narcolepsy. The EEG is normal in both conditions but shows signs of sleep throughout. It is the heavy sleeping which may lead to diagnostic confusion.

Hysterical attacks

Hysteria is a condition in which fits, faints or falls may occur and so again there may be diagnostic difficulty. One of the greatest problems in discussing hysteria is the misunderstanding which this word creates. The doctor uses it to describe a definite psychological disturbance, while a layman may use it merely for an emotional outburst. Some patients with hysteria do exhibit the dramatic behaviour familiar to the layman, for example, floods of tears one moment, and then happy laughter the next. Hysterical symptoms indeed often occur without these dramatic outbursts. In the medical sense the person who suffers from hysteria may lose her voice or develop weakness of the arm or leg. These are called "negative symptoms", while there are also "positive symptoms" which may take the form of an attack. These always happen in the presence of an audience. The patient may lash out at a passer-by, but during the whole of the attack consciousness is not lost, nor does the patient hurt himself, or fall into a deep sleep after the attack. In spite of these obvious differences, fits and hysterical attacks may sometimes closely mimic one another. However, "grande hysteria" is much less common than in the days of Charcot, a Parisian neurologist who first named the condition. His fame was such that doctors flocked from all over Europe to see his clinical demonstrations of patients with neurological disorders. Young and still unknown, Sigmund Freud was among those who made the pilgrimage to Paris.

One advantage the twentieth-century physician has over his predecessors is electro-encephalography. The tracing taken during an hysterical attack is normal, but nearly always specific changes occur during an epileptic fit.

Attacks of dizziness

Attacks of dizziness may be difficult to diagnose and can be confused with epileptic seizures. Dizziness can be severe, and might be accompanied by a sensation of rotation. This condition is called vertigo and is a symptom of Ménière's disease. Here, the organs of balance and hearing, both located deep in the ear, are diseased, and vertigo and deafness occur. This condition often affects the middle-aged and was first described by the Frenchman Hyacinth Ménière. During the attacks of Ménière's disease noises in the ear accompany the feeling of rotation, which may be so severe that the patient falls. These extremely incapacitating attacks often recur every few days. They are generally quite distinct from epilepsy and the E E G is usually normal. In addition, it is rare for epileptic fits to be accompanied by either a feeling of rotation or by any deterioration of hearing.

Drop attacks

The name "drop attack" describes a condition, particularly common in children, in which the patient falls unconscious to the ground. This is, in fact, a form of epilepsy. However, there is a second type of drop attack in which there is a sudden weakness of the legs, so that the patient falls to his knees, but consciousness is preserved and the characteristic pallor of the face during a faint is absent. The predisposing cause is disease in the arteries at the base of the brain. The blood supply in this part becomes insufficient and a series of symptoms occur. The patients may see double, or sight may fade altogether in addition to the unsteadiness and weakness of the legs responsible for the fall. Usually these attacks are recurring, but they are brief and are not convulsive in nature. The E E G may be abnormal, but the disturbance seen is quite different from that observed in patients with epilepsy.

Migraine

It may seem surprising that migraine and epilepsy can be confused, for a fit and a headache are quite dissimilar. However, sometimes the line that separates the two is thin, particularly as attacks in both conditions come "out of the blue". It was Sir William Gowers who in his book *The Borderland of Epilepsy* emphasised the difficulties which may arise. Gowers lived from 1845 to 1915 and was a distinguished British neurologist who contributed greatly to the study of epilepsy and related disorders. Like Hughlings Jackson, he worked at the National Hospital and incidentally gave his name to a mixture used in the treatment of migraine as well as other neurological disorders.

Sometimes when an attack of migraine is severe the patient may faint, while some patients with epilepsy suffer from brief attacks not dissimilar to faints. Again, in some people with epilepsy, a headache or other sensation in the head may precede an epileptic attack, and so there may be confusion with migraine. Just occasionally, however, the patient may have both migraine and epilepsy together, a finding confirmed by Dr Barolin, who wrote in 1966 of a study he had carried out on fifteen thousand patients who attended a neurological centre in

Vienna over the previous few years. He noted that fifteen had epilepsy and migraine together, 570 had epilepsy alone, and 260 had migraine alone. He confirmed that both epilepsy and migraine may be associated with fainting attacks and that, in patients with both disorders, treatment with anti-convulsants and ergot preparations (for migraine) were needed.

Faints and falls form an interesting group of conditions which must be distinguished from epilepsy. To this end X-ray examinations, blood tests and EEGs may be required. Usually, but not always, it is then possible to make a definite diagnosis. Every doctor can recall instances, however, in which he has failed to realise that his patient suffers from epilepsy and also instances in which fits have been diagnosed wrongly. Just occasionally, to confuse matters further, a patient may even simulate epilepsy—Rudyard Kipling wrote of such a one in his poem "The Post that Fitted". Epilepsy, like other conditions, presents a variety of faces.

CHAPTER SIX

What can the doctor do?

THE OCCURRENCE of fits and the subsequent diagnosis of epilepsy is extremely upsetting to the patient as well as to his relatives. Both feel justifiably worried, because epilepsy still carries a stigma in the eyes of the public. However, the aim of the doctor is to help the patient and his family to adjust their lives to this new difficulty. The epileptic sufferer has a handicap, but adjustment is possible, and though he must accept some limitations, these need not be too restrictive. The emphasis should be on what can be done rather than on what cannot.

What to do when a fit occurs

The sight of a person having a convulsive fit can be disturbing, even to trained nurses and doctors, so it is understandable that a layman should be distressed at the sight of a fit in the street. Nevertheless, everyone should have some knowledge of the first aid that is required. First and foremost the patient should be prevented from injuring himself. His head should be supported so that he does not bang it on the ground, and if possible turned to one side to allow the saliva to flow out. Hard objects should be cleared away so that during the jerking phase of the attack the patient does not hit himself against them. In the home he

50

should be taken well away from electric heaters or open fires. Tight clothing, such as a tie or belt, should be loosened to make breathing easier. In the past great store has been set on the insertion of an object into the mouth to prevent injury to tongue and teeth. However, this manœuvre, especially in the rigid or tonic phase of a convulsive attack, is extremely difficult, and no attempt should be made forcefully to insert a hard object. The danger of the patient swallowing his tongue and becoming asphyxiated is greatly overemphasised, and the bystander who is taken unawares need not feel unduly concerned if he cannot carry out any first aid at all, because, though serious injuries do occur, they are rare and death during an attack is most uncommon. In the recovery phase, if the epileptic person is confused and behaves oddly, this should be treated nonchalantly to help prevent embarrassment.

Quite often a person who is subject to fits will have a card (figure 13) or wrist-strap stating this, a fact not as widely known as it should be. Such a card or tag will usually indicate who should be contacted and where the patient should be sent. Someone who has an attack in the street should not be sent immediately to hospital, nor need a doctor necessarily be called. The patient will often recover sufficiently to be able to walk away; if not, he can be taken home in a taxi by a bystander or relative. The disturbance to the epileptic person of being sent into hospital every time he has a fit cannot be overemphasised. However, there are certain circumstances in which an epileptic patient should be seen by his doctor after the occurrence of a single fit, for example if the fit has been much more prolonged and different in character than the usual fits. A doctor should also be called if several fits occur one after the other.

A parent or relative familiar with the patient's attacks will often become aware of the early features of the attack, perhaps a turning of the head to one side. When this occurs the patient can be gently lowered to the floor and put out of reach of hard objects. Often a child having a *petit mal* attack requires no particular treatment, and it is best not to draw attention to them. Occasionally, however, a child may fall during such a fit,

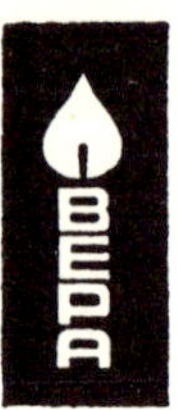

I HAVE EPILEPSY

**Sometimes called fits
or convulsions**

If I should be found unconscious this is NOT because I have been drinking but more probably because I have just had an epileptic attack.

Issued by the
BRITISH EPILEPSY ASSOCIATION, 3-6 Alfred Place, London, W.C.1

My name is..

Address...

.... *Tel.:*..

Nearest Relative....

If I should have a fit, please do not move me unless I am in danger, but leave a clear space around me, loosen my collar, and put something soft under my head. **DO NOT** restrict my movements, **DO NOT** give me anything to drink, **DO NOT** lift me up.

It is not necessary to call an ambulance, the police, or a doctor unless I do not recover consciousness in a few minutes.

I usually recover consciousness in....................minutes.

I am under the care of:

....(doctor or hospital)

....

.... Tel.:....................

FIG. 13. This is a card issued by the British Epilepsy Association and carried by epileptic patients who may have attacks in the street. It indicates to the first aider what he should do for the patient. This kind of card is also carried by diabetics and others on special forms of medication.

52

so if he is standing when an attack occurs a careful watch should be kept. Sometimes the doctor will ask a relative or parent to record every fit to check if they are increasing in number. This also allows assessment of a new medication.

Fits which are followed by confusion, or are accompanied by automatisms, are more difficult to manage, as restraint applied to someone in a state of incomplete awareness may lead to his becoming aggressive. A confused person can be steered more easily from the side than from directly in the front. If he is watched during an epileptic attack so that he can be kept from danger, this should be sufficient and nothing more need be done.

What can the patient be allowed to do?

Care of the patient during an attack represents a very small part of his treatment; organisation of his daily life is perhaps the most important aspect. Parents should handle their children as normally as possible. The child should be encouraged to take part in ordinary school activities, including games, though it is wise to prevent him from climbing ropes in the school gym or riding a bicycle, unless his attacks are well under control. Swimming also presents a problem, but a watchful parent on the side of the swimming-pool will often be sufficient if the child has attacks only seldom and is receiving his medicine regularly. It is true that during games at school the epileptic youth may suffer an injury, but this risk is not much greater than for his non-epileptic colleague, unless he has frequent fits. The emotional effect of prohibiting such activities as football would have to be weighed against the benefits of pursuing such a sport; as in adult life, so in school, idleness and frequent rests are commoner causes of fits than exertion and concentration.

For the adult patient there is no reason why he should not perform an ordinary job. There are certain things, of course, he may not do, such as drive a car or motor-cycle. Ladders and climbing jobs are also forbidden for most, and obviously for patients who have major fits there is danger with machinery.

However, for the patient who has an attack with a warning, or an attack in which one of his limbs jerks but he remains completely conscious throughout, there is no reason why an engineering job cannot be carried out safely and capably. There are many organisations, both privately organised and Government-sponsored, which help in the placing of people with epilepsy in suitable employment (see chapter XIV). Activity is known to discourage fits, so an epileptic patient should engage in physical and mental activity. It is true that excessive fatigue should be discouraged, but it is more important that taking naps in the daytime should be carefully avoided. The EEG shows epileptic activity during relaxation and drowsiness, and in the early stages of sleep, so it is quite possible that a nap during the day might result in a fit. Open air pursuits are excellent, though activities in which head injuries are a risk, like horse riding, should not be undertaken.

There is no reason why a patient with epilepsy should not have a general anaesthetic for a surgical operation or tooth extraction, if this is needed. The only proviso is that the anaesthetist should be informed that the patient has fits and takes anti-epileptic tablets. It is most important that the patient should take his anti-epileptic tablets regularly, and if the administration is not possible in tablet form, injections should be given. Some doctors recommend that children and adults suffering from epilepsy should only receive vaccinations and immunisation if these are essential.

Anti-convulsants

The basis of medical treatment of the person with epilepsy is the use of anti-convulsant tablets.

Bromide was the first drug shown to be effective in controlling epileptic seizures. It came to be introduced, as so often happens with potent remedies, through totally inaccurate reasoning. In 1857 Sieveking read a paper on epilepsy at a medical gathering on his experiments with bromide and Sir Charles Locock commented in the discussion that followed on his cure using the same drug, of thirteen out of fourteen women with epileptic fits occurring at the time of their menstrual periods. Locock apparently had not thought of it as a remedy for all patients with epilepsy, and it was for Wilks to make the remedy popular. Brown-Séquard, another neurologist at the time, also prescribed bromide for convulsive disorders, and interestingly enough in 1861 Hughlings Jackson wrote one of his earliest papers on the treatment of epilepsy by bromide.

In 1912 Alfred Hauptmann in Germany published his first paper on the use of luminal, now called phenobarbitone. Though bromide was effective in some patients, its use was limited because of its side effects. Luminal, however, marked the beginning of a new era in the treatment of epilepsy, as it was a safe and really effective drug. Not until 1939, when Merritt and Putnam in the United States introduced phenytoin, did the next really efficacious drug become available. We were, however, to wait until 1946 for the introduction of troxidone by Richards and Perlstein, the first effective drug for patients with *petit mal* epilepsy. Co-operative research between doctors and chemists has yielded new anti-convulsant medications, but unfortunately the last five years have been almost devoid of progress in this respect.

Both patients and parents become alarmed when daily medication for many months or even for years is suggested by a doctor; but fortunately these anti-convulsant medicines in the proper dosage very rarely lead to unpleasant side effects.

Sometimes patients or their relatives ask whether controlling fits is necessarily a good thing. They suggested that if the brain discharges do not manifest themselves as fits, they may 'come out' in other ways even less acceptable than fits. There is no evidence whatever for such a view. On the contrary, probably the better the fits are controlled, the better the person feels.

When a patient suffers mainly from convulsive fits, either phenytoin or phenobarbitone is usually prescribed. For psycho-motor attacks, phenytoin and primidone, in combination, are often prescribed. *Petit mal* normally requires a rather different kind of medication. Either ethosuximide or troxidone are usually first suggested, though phenobarbitone is sometimes prescribed in combination with these other drugs. (The drugs, their dosage and possible side effects, are listed in detail on pp. 61–7.) A few patients with very infrequent attacks do not need anti-convulsant drugs at all, but this can be decided on only after careful consideration of the particular circumstances.

To obtain full benefit, anti-convulsants must be taken regularly in the prescribed dosage. Usually one tablet, but sometimes two, have to be taken two or even three times a day. They must never be discontinued without a doctor's permission. An abrupt withdrawal of anti-convulsants may lead to *status epilepticus*. In the case of children, tablets will obviously be given by a parent, but adolescents and adults must form regular habits of carrying midday dosages, if required, to school or work. It is particularly important that during holidays or on business trips an adequate supply of tablets or a suitable prescription is available. The anti-convulsant tablets should be regarded by the patient as his friend rather than his enemy, and the doctor can usually foster this attitude by adjusting the dosage and type of tablet carefully.

Anti-convulsant medications are made by many different pharmaceutical manufacturers, and consequently often vary in shape, size and colour of tablet or capsule, even though they contain the same basic medication; and an epileptic patient can become alarmed if he has previously been receiving capsules and then obtains another supply of anti-convulsants in tablet form. Another source of difficulty springs from the fact that some anti-convulsant tablets and capsules contain different mixtures of drugs.

Sometimes, especially when a new treatment is tried, unpleasant symptoms such as drowsiness or dizziness may be noted. These side effects may diminish with time, though on some occasions the new medication may have to be reduced or discontinued. On extremely rare occasions more severe reactions to medication may occur, requiring treatment in hospital. The response to all medications, especially anti-convulsants, varies with the individual, and therefore cannot be predicted. But some drugs have been found to affect many people in the same way. For example, patients complain of unsteadiness and minor stomach upsets after first taking primidone. This medication is therefore started cautiously, and it is usually found that any unpleasant effects gradually pass off. Swelling of the gums, particularly with children, occurs with phenytoin. This looks unpleasant but does not damage the teeth. It is essential that teeth are cleaned regularly, for if the teeth and gums are unhealthy the anti-convulsant is more likely to cause this gum swelling. Regular dental inspection is, of course, necessary.

Regular surveillance

Visits to the doctor's surgery or out-patient department of the local hospital will be necessary to ensure that adequate treatment is being given. Regular checks of the EEG, and sometimes blood tests, may also be required.

Factors causing more fits

Certain conditions may increase the frequency of epileptic attacks. A person who has seizures may learn of these himself and how to avoid them. Irregular taking of anti-convulsant tablets has already been mentioned as a cause of increases in fits. Another is emotional stress; though this may be a factor in adult life, it is often more noticeable in childhood and adolescence. For example, a child who has only a few *petit mal* attacks during the holidays may have an increasing number when he returns to school. Fatigue and lack of sleep may in some susceptible individuals lead to an increase in epileptic attacks. In women at the time of their menstrual periods some increase in the number of fits is often noted. Sometimes during pregnancy attacks may disappear altogether; sometimes they may become more marked. Constipation, influenza and colds may lead to an increase in epileptic attacks. The particular precipitant for fits varies for a given individual, and in some people there appears to be no particular precipitant.

What can the doctor do?

The action of anti-convulsants

Anti-convulsants are not sedatives or tranquillisers; though their action is not entirely understood, they apparently limit the spread of abnormal electrical discharges in the brain and therefore prevent fits. They seem to do this by a special action, not just by general depression of the brain, and, because of this more specific action, do not usually cause drowsiness or other unpleasant side effects. In addition they are not habit-forming, which is clearly a great relief to the epileptic patient.

In most instances treatment, even of mild and infrequent attacks, must be prolonged. Some doctors may even treat for 2–4 years a person who has had a single fit. It should be borne in mind that people with conditions other than epilepsy must take regular medication for many years, for example those with diabetes, pernicious anaemia and some forms of heart disease. In these instances it may be necessary for the medication to be continued for life. So in fact the epileptic patient is in a better position.

Unfortunately anti-convulsants do not "cure" epilepsy, though they do usually control fits. However, in most patients the tendency is for fits to become less frequent as they get older. The hope is that fits are stopped while the patient is on anti-convulsant tablets and that as the tablets are slowly withdrawn the epileptic attacks will not recur. This may be attempted after the patient has had no fits for two or three years, and even then the tablets are only slowly withdrawn over the following year or so. The patient is all this time under medical supervision to make sure there is no recurrence of fits, and his E E G is regularly checked. For about two-thirds, fits will stop altogether, and for the remainder fits will become much less frequent. In addition, almost every year a new medication becomes available, as we have already mentioned, and after careful tests these are tried on those whose attacks still occur on the well tried anti-convulsants. So even if attacks continue, hope should never be lost.

Hormone treatment

In some infants suffering from the disorder known as "infantile spasms", injections of the hormone ACTH are used instead of anti-convulsants. These injections are given perhaps twice a day in a course lasting a few weeks. Attacks are often controlled by this form of treatment, particularly if it is given soon after the disorder commences, but mental retardation cannot apparently be prevented. Unfortunately this hormone treatment is not effective for adults who have fits.

Status epilepticus

Status epilepticus is a serious condition requiring hospital treatment. The patient needs considerable nursing care because he is unconscious and can neither eat nor drink. In addition he requires an anti-convulsant drug. Nowadays diazepam is the first choice, and this is given by injection into a vein so that it can reach the brain more quickly and effectively control the epileptic discharges. Previously paraldehyde was used. Unfortunately, even with the most skilful treatment, a number of such patients die.

Other methods of treatment

Other methods of treatment have been suggested for epilepsy. One of the best known is a special diet, used particularly in the United States, and based on the production of a chemical state in the blood called acidosis. This may occur in patients with diabetes, but also in the normal person as a result of fasting. It explains perhaps the interesting biblical reference to epilepsy which ends with the comment that these attacks "come forth by nothing but prayer and fasting". The epileptic patient after a brief fast is given a diet rich in fats which produces the required acidosis. Unfortunately the diet is unpleasant as well as expensive, and in children it may retard growth. Another drawback is that the control of attacks is unpredictable, and so the treatment is now rarely recommended, though in the past it was useful, when drugs were less effective than they are at present.

What can the doctor do?

Sometimes psychological methods are used in the treatment of epilepsy, either in the form of psychotherapy or hypnosis. Both of these are directed mainly at relieving the patient of the anxieties caused by his incorrect beliefs and fears concerning epilepsy. Hypnosis may, by lowering the level of emotional tension in some individuals, prove a great help, while in others the treatment of emotional difficulties through psychotherapy is more effective. The control of fits requires a combination of these forms of treatment with anti-convulsant tablets. It is completely useless to expect psychological methods alone to control epilepsy.

Unorthodox treatment

Another problem is the desperate search by a parent or relative for unorthodox cures. This may happen if for some reason the patient or his relatives lose faith in their doctor. Non-medical "healers" may be able to help the patient, but sometimes they stop the patient's anti-convulsant drugs and status epilepticus may occur.

Another unfortunate trend, though not permitted in Britain, is the care of the epileptic patient through the post. Diagnosis as well as treatment is surprisingly carried out by "mail order", which is clearly not only inadequate but dangerous. Nevertheless, it does occur, for various reasons. The epileptic patient may, above all, want to avoid having to let the local community know that he has fits. He may fear that the doctor who sees him in his local town will not keep secret the fact that he has epilepsy; hence he may write to a firm in a different city and obtain treatment. In addition, he may think that this treatment is cheaper than attending his local doctor or hospital. Sometimes, however, large fees are extracted from epileptic patients for very inferior service.

The Epilepsy Foundation in Washington D.C. published a pamphlet entitled *Quackery's Gray Area: Mail Order Treatment of Epilepsy*, to emphasise the dangers of this procedure. (In the late nineteenth century, cures for many illnesses, including cancer, syphilis and tuberculosis, were advertised, a practice which is now no longer allowed.) However, according to the pamphlet the practice of treating epilepsy by mail order is conducted in America by at least three firms, none of which is a well-known ethical drug manufacturer. Information about the treatment of epilepsy is offered free on request in certain magazines and then a questionnaire is sent to the patient without his asking. On the basis of this, a diagnosis is made and treatment prescribed. Phenobarbitone is the drug mainly used by these firms, and though this is effective, it should be taken under medical supervision in order to obtain the greatest benefit and avoid side effects, something that is clearly impossible by letter alone.

In summary, the treatment of the patient with epilepsy has two main aspects: the general organisation of his life and the use of anti-convulsant medication. The patient in many instances then improves. However, anti-convulsant medication is unfortunately not curative; only surgery can be, in exceptional cases.

Anti-convulsant medications for major attacks, or temporal lobe attacks

Phenobarbitone. Phenobarbitone (Phenobarbitol, luminal) is perhaps the most widely used anti-convulsant and is usually prescribed in the form of a tablet. The tablets are small and white and contain a variety of dosages. Most commonly used are those containing 30 mgms ($\frac{1}{2}$ grain) or 60 mgms (1 grain) of the substance. One tablet is usually taken two or three times a day. Phenobarbitone is also available in the form of an injection if the patient is suffering from status epilepticus.

This medication is extremely safe. Only rarely do skin rashes occur and they, like the other side effects of phenobarbitone, are seldom serious. Sometimes drowsiness may occur but it does not usually persist. Occasionally a child or adolescent on phenobarbitone may suffer from gross overactivity with extreme irritability. This idiosyncrasy cannot usually be overcome by a reduction of the dosage, which has to be discontinued slowly under doctor's orders, replacing it with another anti-convulsant. In older patients, depression may occur with phenobarbitone, and this too usually requires withdrawal of the drug. Particularly with phenobarbitone gradual replacement with some other medicine is essential to prevent frequent fits.

Newer forms of phenobarbitone have been produced, such as methylpheno-barbitone (mephobarbital), which are marketed under various trade names. These too are usually white tablets containing 200 mgms of the drug. They are taken normally once or twice a day, or sometimes in a single dose at night.

Phenytoin. Phenytoin (Epanutin, Diphenylhydantoin, Dilantin) is a widely used, effective drug produced both in capsule and tablet form. Each is made in two strengths, 50 mgms ($\frac{3}{4}$ grain) or 100 mgms ($1\frac{1}{2}$ grains). Injections of phenytoin are also available for the treatment of patients with status epilepticus.

This drug may lead to a number of side effects, which are, however, rarely dangerous. The most common is swelling of the gums, unpleasant in appearance but treatable by the dentist. The gum swelling is unlikely to occur if the teeth are brushed regularly and gums are free from infection. Sometimes rashes which may be confused with measles occur in association with enlargement of glands in the armpits or elsewhere in the body. Occasionally a patient will complain of unsteadiness in walking. Such a state of affairs may occur at the beginning of treatment or if the patient is receiving a heavy dose of medicine. Drowsiness is uncommon with phenytoin, but in a few patients anaemia may appear after many years of medication.

Primidone. Primidone (Mysolin) completes the triad of better-known drugs for the treatment of major epilepsy. In Britain this is available as a white tablet, lined and marked with the manufacturer's initials. Each tablet contains 250 mgms of the anti-convulsant. For the treatment of children there are smaller tablets and it is also available in liquid form.

Primidone has a number of well-recognised side effects. These occur especially at the beginning of the course of treatment.

The patient may complain of unsteadiness and possibly drowsiness. The side effects pass if the dose is maintained at the same level and subsequently, even with an increasing dose of primidone, they do not usually recur. Serious side effects are very unusual. Primidone is closely related to phenobarbitone.

For minor attacks

Ethosuximide. Ethosuximide (Zarontin) is now generally the first choice for the treatment of *petit mal* epilepsy; it is available as capsules containing an orange-coloured liquid, or as tablets. Both contain 250 mgms of the substance and are usually taken one to three times a day.

Ethosuximide is remarkably free from unpleasant side effects but sometimes the patient may complain of headaches or drowsiness, or occasionally of mental slowness and confusion.

Troxidone. Troxidone (tridione, trimethadione) is made in the form of capsules containing 300 mgms of the active substance. Usually one or two capsules are taken three times a day. This drug, which in the past was the only one available for the treatment of *petit mal,* may have fairly serious side effects in some patients. The most common is known as the glare phenomenon, which is the name used to describe a snowstorm effect which the patient sees in his field of vision. Unfortunately, reduction of the dose of the drug does not usually help. Sometimes patients may complain of double vision and skin rashes may be encountered, as well as joint pains and fevers. Serious blood disorders may also occur. These are described under methoin (see below).

Other anti-convulsants used in the treatment of epilepsy

Bromide. Bromide was the first effective anti-convulsant medication, but it is now very rarely used, because it is not as simple to administer as the modern anti-epileptic drugs. It may be prescribed in a variety of forms, either tablet or liquid. Bromide tends to accumulate in the body and, in fact, gradually replaces an essential constituent of the blood known as chloride. Frequent checks of the blood to ascertain how much bromide is present are therefore necessary.

A wide variety of side effects occur. Sometimes, especially in young children and adolescents, acne-like rashes occur which are very difficult to treat. The patient often complains of drowsiness, particularly in hot weather, and there is marked perspiration and loss of chloride from the body. Less commonly patients on bromide develop serious nervous disorders. These can almost always be corrected by withdrawal of bromide and by replacement with another anti-convulsant.

Ethotoin. Ethotoin (peganone) is prepared as 500 mgms tablets. One or two of these tablets are taken two or three times a day. This drug has similar side effects to phenytoin.

Methoin. Methoin (mesantoin, mephenytoin) is administered as 100 mgms tablets taken two or three times a day; unfortunately this drug, although particularly effective in patients with temporal lobe epilepsy, has many serious side effects. It is now therefore less frequently used, particularly because of its tendency to cause blood disorders.

These blood disorders have been reported with a variety of anti-epileptic drugs apart from methoin. They also occur with other medicines used in the treatment of many diseases. The blood consists of a fluid containing salt and other substances in solution as well as solid elements. These elements are the red blood cells which carry oxygen and the white blood cells which defend the body against infectious organisms. These two types of cells are made mainly by the bone marrow which is located in the hollow spaces in the limb and other bones. Drugs may suppress the bone marrow and as a result it is unable to make the correct number of cells. The number circulating in the blood is diminished. Anti-convulsant medications sometimes suppress the production of the white cells, a condition which is known as agranulocytosis. As a result resistance to infection is diminished. Aplastic anaemia is a disturbance in which the production of both red and white cells is suppressed.

Phenylacetylurea. Phenylacetylurea (pheneurone, phenacemide) is supplied in the form of white tablets containing 500 mgms of the anti-convulsant substance. One or two of these tablets are usually prescribed up to three times a day. Unfortunately, this substance may in rare instances have extremely toxic effects, especially on the liver and the blood as in the case of methoin. Hence, though it is effective it is used less frequently than other medications. It is also marketed in combination with pheno-barbitone.

Paramethadione (paradione). This drug is similar to troxidone and is also used for patients with *petit mal.*

Sulthiame. Sulthiame (ospolot) has only recently become available. These tablets contain 200 mgms of the active substance, and one or two are prescribed two or three times a day. This medication is effective in temporal lobe epilepsy. Fairly frequent minor side effects are reported by the patients when they take this medicine. They develop tingling in the hands and sometimes rapid breathing. Oddly enough, in the patients who have these side effects, the drug is often more effective in controlling attacks, and sometimes these unpleasant symptoms pass.

Carbamazepine (tegretol). This is prepared as tablets containing 200 mgms of the effective substance and one or two are taken two or three times a day. It is favoured by many doctors as the drug of choice in temporal lobe epilepsy. It can, however, cause blood disorders.

Additional medications sometimes used in the treatment of epilepsy

Acetazolamine. Acetazolamine (diamox) is available in the form of a white tablet which contains 250 mgms of the active substance. This substance is a diuretic (which means it leads to an increased production of urine) and was introduced because it was observed that fluid may be retained in the body just before the menstrual flow begins in women. Fits have also been observed to be frequent in some patients at that time. Acetazolamine has also been found to be effective in other forms of epilepsy. Possible side effects are that it may sometimes cause tingling in the limbs, and in some patients nausea and vomiting.

Amphetamine. This drug, marketed under a variety of trade names, is occasionally used in the treatment of epilepsy. The tablets usually contain 5 mgms of the active substance and one to four may be taken per day. It is sometimes used for patients on large doses of other anti-convulsant medication that have made them drowsy and lacking in energy. It is also an effective anti-convulsant in its own right.

The side effects of amphetamine are fairly frequent; it can lead to loss of appetite and weight and sometimes inability to sleep at night. In some patients it may cause irritability and restlessness during the day.

Chlordiazepoxide (librium). This drug is marketed in the form of capsules or tablets. These contain either 5 or 10 mgms of the active substance. This medicine which is well known as a tranquilliser has been used for epileptic patients. Usually one tablet is given two or three times a day. On first taking this drug the patient may feel mildly unsteady on his feet. A feeling of drowsiness has been reported too but only very rarely.

Diazepam (valium). This drug is manufactured in a variety of sizes and colours of tablets, depending on whether the tablet contains 2 mgms, 5 mgms or 10 mgms of the active substance. It is also available as an injection. This substance is similar to chlordiazepoxide in action and is used as a long-term treatment for epileptic patients. However, it has been discovered to be of particular value in the treatment of status epilepticus, when it is administered by injection. Nitrazepam (mogadon) is a compound related to diazepam and has been used in the treatment of infantile spasms. Clonazepam, another substance in the same series, is a recent addition and not yet generally available. It is said to be useful for the long-term treatment of most types of epilepsy.

Two other substances, not strictly anti-convulsant medicines, are effective in the treatment of very select groups of young patients with epileptic attacks.

The first is *pyridoxine* or vitamin B$_6$. Some infants whose food is lacking in this vitamin may have many fits, and if it is then added to their diet the number of fits will decrease markedly. It is, however, very rarely effective in the treatment of adult epilepsy.

Another preparation which has been used in the treatment of infants with "infantile spasms" is ACTH. This hormone is given in a course lasting a few weeks and is sometimes effective in reducing the number of attacks. Unfortunately this treatment is less effective than was at first thought and it has no place in the control of epilepsy in adults.

An International Glossary. The International Bureau for Epilepsy (see p. 136) has now published an excellent glossary of anti-convulsants which gives the names for equivalent preparations all over the world. This is of course particularly useful for people moving permanently to other countries or staying for prolonged periods, as well as for foolhardy holiday-makers who leave their two or three weeks supply of anti-convulsants on the bedside table.

CHAPTER SEVEN

What can the surgeon do?

NEUROSURGICAL operations are older than the word epilepsy itself. Trephining, or the removal of a small piece of the skull, was performed as early as the Stone Age. Why the operation was carried out is not known; could it have been to treat epilepsy? Probably not—it is much more likely that it was done to allow 'evil spirits' to escape!

Not until the end of the nineteenth century did the modern era of brain surgery begin. Sir Victor Horsley was among the most important contributors to this renaissance when he introduced the operation known as a craniotomy. In this operation, a piece of skull bone is removed to reveal the membraneous coverings of the brain underneath. These are cut and turned aside so that the underlying cortex or outer surface of the brain can be seen. On 25 May 1886 Sir Victor performed his first craniotomy in the presence of Hughlings Jackson. The patient was a twenty-two-year-old Scotsman who at the age of fifteen had suffered a head injury, since when he had had very frequent focal attacks starting from the brain scar that occurred when his skull was fractured. The scar was removed from the brain surface and his seizures ceased.

Indications for operation

Unfortunately this operation is possible for only a very few people with epilepsy, for two main reasons. The first concerns the type of epilepsy. At present only forms of epilepsy arising in a discrete area of brain—focal epilepsy—are suitable. Generalised types, in which the basic defect is probably a widespread inability of the cells of the nervous system to limit the spread of epileptic discharge, are unsuitable.

The second reason why an operation is not always possible concerns the location of the abnormality. If a brain scar is near a vital area of the brain, for example that concerned with speech or movement of the limbs, operation may result in loss of speech (aphasia) or paralysis of part of the body.

Neurosurgical centres

The complicated series of tests that are required to select patients for the surgical treatment of epilepsy are usually carried out in special centres. The surgeon must be sure, first of all, that there is a definite scar in the brain and, as far as it is possible, only one such scar. In addition, he has to check that such an abnormality is the cause of the fits and that it is in a site that he can reach and remove without severe damage to the brain. This clearly is a considerable undertaking, and special teams of investigators are collected in certain centres in the world to carry out the investigations and evaluate the results of their operative treatment of the patients. Such techniques are time consuming and expensive—more reasons why such operations are performed relatively seldom. The number and variety of tests are changing as refinements are made and new methods are introduced. Some of the tests used most widely will now be described.

Special EEG tests

Many EEGs have to be performed in order to make sure that

there is only one diseased area, for example that the left temporal lobe is scarred while the right temporal lobe is healthy. An important procedure for determining this involves the injection of pentylenetetrazol, an agent that may cause a fit. The E E G is recorded while this substance is slowly injected. (Pentylenetetrazol is not given quickly, as this may produce a sudden major convulsive fit which does not help the surgeon as he would not then be able to ascertain where the attack started; he wants to find the site of the first epileptic discharge.) As the injection continues the patient may experience a twitch at the corner of the mouth or a tingling sensation in the arm. The injection is stopped till this has been accurately described and the electrical charges in the E E G examined. The injection is begun again and continued till the patient has his habitual fit.

In order to analyse the pattern of the attack more accurately a film is often taken, as well as a tape-recording of the patient's and doctor's descriptions of the attack, how it began and the way it developed. The combination is often vital in deciding whether or not the fit began in one area of the brain and whether or not this could be treated by an operation.

Another preliminary investigation is called "depth recording". An operation is carried out in which a small piece of the skull bone is removed. Through this hole, at the same operation, fine wire electrodes are inserted into that part of the brain which is thought, from other tests, to be responsible for starting the fit. Detailed E E G recordings with these special depth electrodes can then be carried out over several days if necessary, to make certain of the site or origin of the epileptic discharges.

Other special tests

Special X-ray tests are performed on some patients with epilepsy, as described in chapter IV. These are particularly necessary if surgery is contemplated, and from them it is usually possible to make a confident prediction about the site, for example a scar in the brain. However, unlike the E E G, it is not possible to tell from an X-ray whether a revealed abnormality is the source of the epileptic discharge which causes the patient's fits.

Another type of test is carried out by the psychologist, who also works in the neurosurgical centre. Particular psychological functions are located in certain areas of the brain. For example, the temporal lobe on the left side is concerned with complicated hearing and speech mechanisms. Special tests have been constructed that can detect which temporal lobe is diseased and may thus aid the surgeon in locating the scar and its extent.

If the evidence from all these different tests shows that there is a single area of damage in the brain which is responsible for fits, then an operation can be undertaken. Even from this brief outline, it will be seen that these preliminaries are complicated, and in addition place a strain on both patient and doctor. For this reason the usual practice is to consider operation only after a thorough trial of all other methods of treatment. This perhaps sounds strange to the layman, who may feel that an operation is the only satisfactory course of action. Unfortunately there is a certain risk in operation and the cure is not always absolute, as we shall see later.

The operation

The operation itself involves the exposure of the brain surface, and it may come as a surprise that this is usually carried out not under a general, but under a local, anaesthetic. The patient is given a sedative as a preliminary, and then the scalp is injected with a local anaesthetic agent which deadens the pain. The brain itself, however, is quite insensitive to pain or touch. The technique clearly requires great confidence in the surgeon from the patient. However, with a local anaesthetic the patient is able to cooperate in the various important manœuvres of the surgeon during the operation.

In the operating theatre, apart from the patient, the nurses, the surgeon and his assistants, is the electro-encephalographer with his apparatus. He has two duties to perform. First he has to record the electrical activity directly from the surface of the brain (the electro-corticogram), instead of from the surface of the scalp (the electro-encephalogram). Secondly, in collaboration with the surgeon, he is responsible for the electrical stimulation apparatus. This is used to stimulate certain areas of

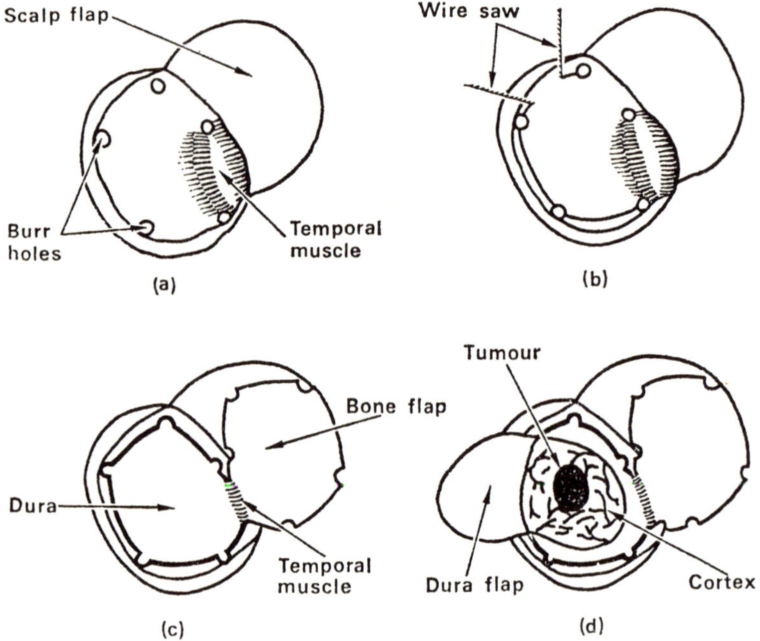

FIG. 14. The sequence of actions carried out by the surgeon to reach the brain.

(a) First the scalp is turned back and small holes drilled in the skull.
(b) A wire saw is inserted from one hole in the skull to the next and then used to saw between the holes. This is repeated several times.
(c) The section of bone is then removed and the meninges covering the brain are exposed.
(d) After the meninges have been turned back the cortex of the brain with the tumour can be seen.

the brain and forms a very important part of the operative procedure. Because it is necessary to elicit the response of the patient to stimulation, a general anaesthetic cannot be used.

When all the apparatus and assistants are ready the operation begins. The surgeon turns aside the scalp and deeper tissues until he reaches the skull bone (figure 16). He then removes a section of the bone over the presumed site of the brain abnormality. Next, he deflects the coverings of the brain so that the meninges and the surface of the brain are exposed. Electrodes are placed on the brain and the electro-encephalographer makes a recording of the brain activity. This confirms, for the surgeon, the localisation of the abnormality diagnosed already by the preliminary tests described. However, the amount of brain tissue actually removed is often determined by electrical stimulation procedures.

Stimulation of the brain

The surgeon warns the patient that he may feel some unusual sensations or movements, and he is asked to describe these as fully as possible. A special electrode is gently placed on the brain surface, and a brief small electrical current is passed through this. If the stimulating electrode is over the brain area responsible for initiating movement of the hand, then the hand may twitch. Because of the arrangement of the fibres in the brain, if the right side of the brain is stimulated it is the left hand which moves, and the same is true with the other areas of the brain. As each stimulation is carried out, the surgeon places a small numbered piece of paper on the surface of the brain so that the various responses can be correlated. A photograph is taken at the end of the stimulation procedure so that a permanent record is made. Usually, in addition, a secretary records the surgeon's comments as he finishes each stimulation.

Before an abnormal piece of tissue is removed from the brain, the area responsible for speech must be located. This must not be damaged or the patient might not be able to speak properly after the operation, so the surgeon asks the patient to repeat a nursery rhyme over and over, and he then stimulates at various points on the surface of the brain; from his previous experience he knows the rough location of this area. The patient suddenly stops saying the nursery rhyme when the point stimulated is over the speech area.

On some occasions stimulation of parts of the temporal lobe leads to vivid recall of complex memories with sights, smells and emotions. This indicates that the temporal lobe is closely concerned with storing memories. These stimulation studies help to clarify the basic mechanisms of the brain as well as of the fits themselves. A focal fit beginning in the temporal lobe may have an aura of a smell preceding the onset, or a complex memory, while a fit beginning in the area responsible for leg movement will merely lead to a jerking of the legs without other more complex behavioural changes.

Sometimes during the operation, the patient may without warning have a fit. This is troublesome if it happens unexpectedly. However, there are times when if the surgeon is still uncertain about the origin of the patient's attack he will actually bring one on during the operation by an injection of a convulsant drug. The site of the epileptic discharge can be determined by the electrical recording from the brain surface during the injection, and this can confirm for us the way epileptic discharges behave in the brain. The localised electrical abnormality corresponds to a focal fit and the quick spreading discharge to the *grand mal*.

Temporal lobectomy

Once the brain stimulation has been done the patient is given a general anaesthetic and surgical removal of brain tissue is carried out. Most frequently it is the tip of the temporal lobe which is excised, as this is one of the commonest sites from which epileptic discharges arise. After the removal of the diseased part of the brain, the covering of the brain and scalp are stitched back into place. Though the operation sounds daunting, patients usually have a smooth recovery.

This operation is carried out in Britain about a hundred times a year.

Results

The results obtained by Wilder Penfield in Canada, Earl Walker in the United States and Murray Falconer in England, to give examples of three surgeons who carry out such operations, are rather similar. About half the patients are completely cured; in about a third of the remaining patients there is a marked diminution in frequency of fits, and in the rest there is little change.

The results may seem surprising, for if an epileptic area of the brain is removed, it might be expected that the cure rate would be 100 per cent. To study this problem further a careful analysis of the part of the brain removed is carried out by the pathologist. Sometimes he reports that there may be other areas of disease elsewhere in the brain, and this view is supported sometimes by the electro-encephalographer's report on EEGs carried out after operations, which show new epileptic areas. Further operations are sometimes carried out, though for many patients this is not possible.

In recent years various surgeons have made new approaches to the treatment of epilepsy, for example by use of computer analysis of "depth recording" (see p. 70) prior to removal of the focal electrical abnormality. Others have devised techniques which would be applicable to those patients who have generalised fits. At the present time, the value of these new techniques, which involve interruption of pathways to prevent the spread of discharges from one part of the brain to another, is not proven. However, as with the type of surgery described in detail already, thorough investigation of the patient and careful assessment of the results is the only way in which we shall determine whether these methods will have a wider application.

CHAPTER EIGHT

Children with fits

EPILEPSY in early life is, as William Lennox said, "more puzzling, more diversified than in adults, a rich field only partially explored".

Fits in infancy present special problems for many reasons. First, the brain of an infant or young child is still developing and so the types of seizure may be different from those seen in an older child. Secondly, fits are often frequent. Thirdly, the developing brain is particularly susceptible to injury and infections. Fourthly, diagnosis is often more difficult and the EEG may be more abnormal than in adults. Fifthly, treatment has a much broader scope, and must involve the whole family situation. In particular, the fear and shame of parents having young children with fits must be dealt with.

Children may have almost every type of fit, but the *petit mal* attack is almost entirely limited to childhood; while *grand mal* attacks are also frequent, temporal lobe attacks are uncommon. However, one kind of attack is special only to the first years of life—"infantile spasms".

Infantile spasms

In 1841 W. J. West, a doctor, published a letter in the *Lancet* about his own child, who had infantile spasms and was in addition suffering from mental subnormality. This was perhaps the first account of this condition, and as Jeavons and Bower said in their assessment of this condition in the *Lancet* of 1956, "these patients remain a burden of hopeless pity for those who care for them".

This condition is widely known throughout the world. It has many names—"Salaam" spasms, massive myoclonic jerks, jack-knife convulsions, lightning spasms, or in German *Blitznick*. It is usually associated with the grossly disorganised EEG pattern known as hypsarrhythmia (see figure 15). These names are used to describe a variety of brief, generalised, sudden attacks. The commonest type of attack is as follows: the arms are flung forwards and out from the trunk, the legs bend at the hips. Sometimes the trunk bends forward and sometimes the head only bends forward as the arms are jerked outwards. Just occasionally only one arm is affected. There may also be a cry associated with the attack.

The attacks can be very frequent and often they occur just before the child goes off to sleep or just on waking. In addition to the "jack-knife" attacks, longer fits not dissimilar to *grand mal* also occur. Infantile spasms affect only very young infants, and most commonly they begin between three months and a year, although they may sometimes occur in children up to three years of age. Boys are affected twice as frequently as girls. In addition to spasms, there is often mental retardation. This is sometimes obvious before the attacks develop but occasionally is only noted afterwards.

Infantile spasms may be the result of brain injury, for example, through a haemorrhage into the brain at birth, or because breathing did not start at once after birth and the brain suffered from lack of oxygen for a short period. Sometimes this condition results when some of the chemical processes which are normally carried out in the body are deranged. The most common and well known of these conditions is phenylketonuria. This particular condition can be detected by the demonstration of an abnormal substance in the urine, and for this reason it is now routine to test the urine of babies soon after birth. In the positive cases a special diet begun at once can prevent spasms or other complications of the condition. Sometimes these spasms begin after immunisation for diphtheria, but in many instances no definite cause can be found. It should be realised that this is a rare condition, though a distressing one, particularly because of

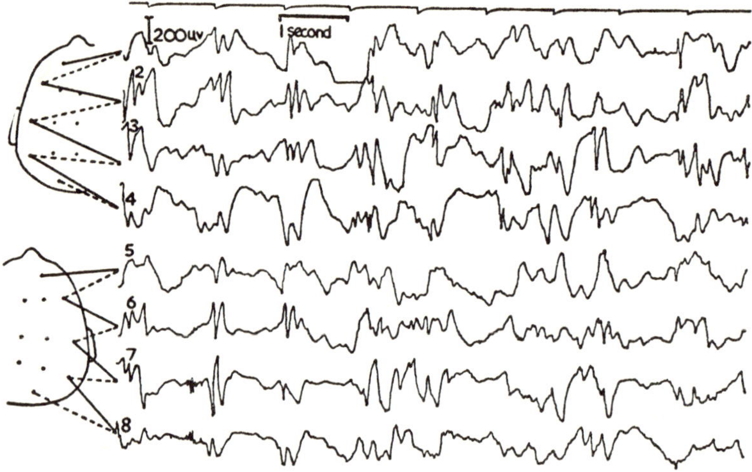

FIG. 15. EEG of a child of five months old showing the typical irregular hypsarrhythmic pattern seen when the patient has infantile spasms.

the associated mental retardation. This persists after the spasms have been replaced by other types of fits.

The EEG is helpful in the diagnosis of infantile spasms, for it is grossly abnormal and quite different from that recorded in other types of epilepsy (figure 15); there is marked irregularitry with many slow waves and spikes. These often come in groups which coincide with the spasm. This characteristic EEG pattern was first described in 1951; seventeen years later Dr Sorel published an enthusiastic report on the therapeutic effect of the hormone ACTH. The report indicated that, when the spasms stopped, the EEG improved and most important of all there was improvement in the mental state of the infant.

Jeavons and Bowers described one hundred and twelve

infants whom they studied over a ten-year period. They tried a variety of hormone preparations including ACTH, at the same time carefully recording the progress of the infants and carrying out repeated EEGs. The spasms stopped completely in seventy of their patients, and in just under half the EEG became normal. Recently nitrazepam (mogadon) has been used with some success in the treatment of this condition, but even so, many of these children continue to have some form of epilepsy, usually major fits. On the whole, therefore, the outlook is rather depressing for these young patients with infantile spasms.

Febrile convulsions

Infants up to the age of five may have convulsions associated with a rise in body temperature. In the past convulsions have been blamed particularly on teething, but very often they accompany a cold, tonsillitis, or almost any infection. Sometimes the doctor may find it a problem to discover the reason for the convulsion, and doubly difficult because a convulsion itself may cause a slight rise in body temperature. As William Lennox noted, "the solution of the cause of the febrile convulsions resembles the best-selling who-done-it". There is no doubt that if a child has an infection, then the causative organisms, be they virus or bacteria, may produce poisons or toxins in the body and these, by their effect on the brain, could lead to a convulsion. This is really more a plausible theory than a proven fact. Like so many areas of epilepsy there is uncertainty and doubt.

The doctor is in a particularly difficult situation, since he must examine the young patient, decide the cause of the convulsion, and in addition consider which treatment if any is indicated. There is great difference of opinion about this; many physicians would in fact dismiss a single convulsion as unimportant, while others would regard such an action as almost amounting to neglect. However, a second convulsion is almost always regarded as serious, and anti-convulsant treatment is started in dosages appropriate for the small size of the child.

There are three signs that suggest the attacks are serious; if they are prolonged, affect one part of the body, for example the left arm and leg, rather than both sides of the body equally, and if the E E G shows an abnormality on one side. When these features are present, the treatment is always begun with anti-convulsants. The medication is usually continued for a year or two and then carefully withdrawn.

Some doctors believe that febrile convulsions occur in those who have epilepsy or febrile convulsions in the family, while others deny this. Again some consider that children with febrile convulsions will have fits as adults, and others deny this. In spite of many studies from all parts of the world uncertainty persists.

Repeated febrile convulsions may sometimes lead to brain damage. Therefore a child who is susceptible to convulsions should have minor illnesses carefully treated as well as receiving anti-convulsant medications. In this way brain damage may be prevented. Fortunately most children who have had febrile convulsions grow up to be healthy and normal adults, free of fits.

Abdominal epilepsy

Abdominal epilepsy is the name given to a curious condition in which the young patient complains of abdominal pain from time to time. Doctors are really not certain about the cause of this condition, or in many instances whether it is a form of epilepsy at all. Sometimes the name "periodic syndrome" or "abdominal migraine" is used. Of course, if the child also suffers from definite fits the diagnosis is easier. On occasions, however, the young patient has just sudden brief attacks of pain in the stomach which last a few hours and are accompanied by a feeling of sickness without vomiting. Sometimes the pain is quite severe, lasts for several days and is associated with fever. Headaches and generalised weakness also occur. The E E G may be abnormal and the conditions respond to anti-convulsant medication. If other members of the family have suffered from headaches or seizures in their youth this is a valuable clue in diagnosis.

At times symptoms occur in tense, anxious children who also have migraine. If there is no definite history of epileptic attacks then they are treated for migraine and anxiety with the usual medicine. If, on the other hand, there are EEG abnormalities of epileptic type and definite fits, anti-convulsants are usually given. This is one of the borderlands of epilepsy and, aping Gertrude Stein, we may say a fit is a fit is a fit, but a stomach ache—usually but not always!

"Hyperkinetic syndrome"

Most children, as every parent knows, are at some stage in their lives overactive; they dart from one interest to another and lack concentration. However, there is a type of overactivity which is more marked by its persistence, its severity and its association with destructive behaviour. This has been labelled the "hyperkinetic syndrome". Oddly enough, though these children are overactive, if they can be persuaded to rest in the middle of the day they fall quickly into a deep sleep—in fact, some doctors have suggested that their sleep is much deeper and less restless than their unaffected brothers and sisters. This particular hyperkinetic syndrome has been described in children whose brain has been damaged, either by infection or head injury, or by the occurrence of severe epileptic attacks. Fortunately the hyperkinetic syndrome, which tends to affect boys rather than girls, passes as the child gets older, so that by the age of nine or ten he is no more distractable, overactive or troublesome than any normal child.

At home parents may tolerate this overactivity, but these children are particularly difficult at school. They may well have to be excluded from their normal school classes to attend a special school. If they can, in spite of everything, receive adequate schooling, they may develop normally. However, the hyperkinetic syndrome is sometimes associated with a mild degree of mental retardation, whether the child has epilepsy or not.

Children with fits

Difficulties of diagnosis

As was said earlier, epilepsy in the young child may present difficulties in diagnosis. This is because there may be many different causes, but also because it is more difficult to carry out the investigations, blood tests, X-rays and EEGs which in an adult would be simple. In addition a number of conditions which lie on the borderland of epilepsy must be differentiated. Breath-holding spells (see p. 45) are one example; another is fainting attacks, which occur in children as well as in adults (see p. 43). They are not particularly common in the very young and become more frequent around puberty, with its various stresses. In the past, nightmares and sleep-walking, if frequent, were coupled with epilepsy, but they are quite unrelated.

To summarise, the baby, the infant, the toddler and the school child can all suffer from some form of epilepsy. In the first year or so of life the baby may suffer "infantile spasms". This, unfortunately, still has no satisfactory form of treatment; apart from this serious condition, many young children who develop epilepsy grow up normally and are schooled with their fellows who are free from fits.

CHAPTER NINE

Do fits affect the mind?

THERE are many misconceptions and half-truths about fits and the people who have them. Perhaps the most important is the belief that the epileptic person is of unstable personality and poor intelligence. There is not much evidence for these beliefs, and such statements are unfortunate because they add a further burden to the sufferer, who already has a genuine disability with which to cope. Fear that he may have an attack at any time is, to say the least, inconvenient and may even cause injury. His disability is inconstant, quite unlike that of a man with deafness, blindness or a wooden leg who is incapacitated, but all the time.

The epileptic subject has genuine difficulties which may generate a constant and understandable sense of insecurity. Coupled with these, as we shall see, are social problems such as finding suitable employment. Even finding suitable accommodation is sometimes beset with difficulties. Despite all this, there are many people with fits who lead active and valuable lives.

In the past, too, there was a constant fear of being put into a hospital or an epileptic colony which again contributed to the feeling of insecurity. Fortunately now, with the introduction of newer and more plentiful anti-convulsant drugs and an improved attitude towards employment and community care, epileptic colonies are barely needed.

The child with epilepsy

Epilepsy, as mentioned already, frequently begins in childhood or early adult life. Clearly such an occurrence affects the parents of the sufferer. Their reaction to epilepsy and the way they handle it will have a profound effect on the child. They have a difficult task in deciding what is best for the child. Sometimes they allow themselves to be brain-washed into believing the very misconceptions that have already been described and we know to be untrue. If they tend to reject the child or are unduly anxious, or treat him as though he has a serious illness, then their attitudes will be transmitted to the child. Over-protection, however, should also be avoided at all costs. It must be decided for each patient whether he may cycle or swim, for example. If the parents do reject their child, he may become belligerent, refuse his anti-convulsant medication, or be deceitful about taking it. Mismanagement of the child, too, may lead to isolation and behaviour problems which would not have occurred if handling had been along common-sense lines.

Normal discipline is required as much for the epileptic child as for his fellows. When there are others in the family, there should be no favouritism for the one with fits. Spoiling in the long run can only lead to greater difficulties. These will, in their turn, limit the patient's ability to adapt to the harder world of adult life without parental blandishments. There are, of course, risks in allowing the child a fairly free life in spite of his attacks, but these are not great and as a result he will gain self-confidence. Harsh restrictions will only lead to frustration. Similarly, the attitude of school teachers to epileptic attacks will aid or detract from the child's educational progress. (Specific problems of education will be dealt with in chapter XIV.)

Whether or not the neighbours should be told of the child's disability is a difficult problem. If they are not, there is, of course, the fear that a fit may occur in the garden or even in the neighbour's house. Secrecy can often lead to greater difficulty and to limitations of the child's normal pursuits and games. If the epilepsy is not well controlled, close supervision is clearly required, and everyone in contact with the child should be encouraged to help with this. But if the fits are infrequent, then constant observation is both unwarranted and harmful. A social worker can help parents with these very real problems.

Is intelligence affected by fits?

Having dealt with the general psychological problems, particularly of the child, it is important to consider intelligence. A group of patients with epilepsy has a range of intelligence quotients from very high to very low, and equal numbers fall in the middle of this range, as in the general population. In the past when epileptic patients, mainly from institutions, had their intelligence assessed by psychologists, there was an excess in the low-normal or sub-normal group. This was due to a sampling error and did not express the true situation. There are lawyers, doctors, businessmen and writers who have fits and who are still very intelligent. Epilepsy is no bar to genius or eccentricity, but equally well, no bar to normality. However, there are two further points here: first, does the occurrence of fits ever damage the brain and lead to deterioration? Patients who have had frequent attacks which have failed to respond to treatment, may deteriorate intellectually, but this is a small minority. On the other hand, William Lennox reported an interesting experiment by nature herself. Pairs of identical twins, one with and one without fits, were examined, and in spite of repeated seizures, there was usually no deterioration in the intelligence in most of the twins with fits as compared with their more fortunate brother or sister.

The second point is this: many children of sub-normal intelligence have epileptic attacks. It is often the case that retardation of development is noted even before the fits start, and thus epilepsy cannot be blamed for the retardation. It seems that

Do fits affect the mind?

both epilepsy and mental retardation are due to a common cause: for example, damage to the child's brain occurring during the mother's pregnancy, at birth, or by illness in the early years of life. Epilepsy, like retardation, is a symptom of the basic condition—brain damage.

Children with fits and retardation often require a great deal of attention and this may not always be possible at home. Many have to be admitted to institutions where they are cared for, and they may have to remain there, unfortunately, for the rest of their lives. Certain rare and specific diseases occur in children that cause low intelligence and epilepsy at the same time. For example, phenylketonuria (already described) and the Sturge-Weber syndrome in which calcium is deposited in the brain.

Is the personality affected by fits?

Sometimes epileptic patients appear slow and dreamy, and it is possible that this is the result of side effects from their anti-convulsant drugs. Phenobarbitone may cause drowsiness some-times. On other occasions it may cause restlessness and on rare occasions depression. Other medications produce similar problems, and these side effects may be the price that the epileptic patient pays in order to have his fits controlled, though such a situation arises much less frequently than in the past because of the increase in the number of medications in the doctor's armamentarium. He can, if the patient develops side effects, change to another drug.

In the early days of the century a specific epileptic per-sonality was described by doctors. The patients were said to be sly, aggressive, impulsive, obsequious, and many other unpleasant adjectives were applied. These epileptic patients spent many years isolated from society, crowded in locked wards and mental hospitals, on repeated doses of drugs which, were much more toxic than the present medications. The older drugs not only led to severe ill-health and death, but also in order to be effective they had to be given in large doses. Such a combination of unpleasant circumstances could easily lead to bizarre personality traits even in non-epileptic people. However, Barbara Tizard recently reviewed many studies concerned with the "epileptic personality" and was unable to find convincing evidence that such a condition existed. So it appears that with more effective treatment the "epileptic personality" has disappeared. Most medical authorities would agree with this conclusion. However, there is conflicting evidence and some doctors feel that a small minority of those with epilepsy do show personality abnormalities. These are usually patients with fits arising in the temporal lobe, and then operation with removal of the epileptic focus may produce beneficial results.

The patients who show a personality disorder are said always to have had fits for many years, and often increasing medication has been administered for a similar period. Slowness and repetitiveness and irritability are regarded as the most noticeable features of this disorder, though, of course, these too may be found in many non-epileptic people.

Mental illness and epilepsy

Depression and neuroses are seen in epileptic patients, but probably no more frequently than in the non-epileptic person. However, concerning the illness of schizophrenic type there are differences of opinion among doctors. Schizophrenia is not frequent in epileptic patients, but it seems that in a minority who have temporal lobe epilepsy it may occur more often than would be expected by chance. In other words, there is an association between a brain disorder and schizophrenia. This is of interest, as most patients with a severe psychosis like schizophrenia have no definite brain disturbance as detected by electrical and other means of investigation during life. In addition, even after a prolonged illness, when the brain is examined at post mortem, no disorder is noted. The number of epileptic patients who develop schizophrenia, however, is very small and they can still be treated with appropriate medication and other methods.

CHAPTER TEN

Epilepsy in history

THE SACRED disease, an ancient name for epilepsy, is probably
the oldest-known disorder of the brain. As early as 2080 BC it
was mentioned in the Hammurabi Laws and then as now had
medico-social importance. The sacred disease was known to
both the ancient Egyptians and the Hebrews. In the Talmud
it was stated that peculiar behaviour of parents during cohabi-
tation could lead to epilepsy in the child. The sacred disease,
therefore, was familiar well before the writings of Hippocrates
about 400 BC.

In Greek, just as in English, one would say of any disease that
it had "seized" a man. This terminology probably derives from
the idea that all diseases were considered to be attacks by gods
or demons, and probably accounts for the name "sacred disease". Thus the whole history of epilepsy is linked with the story
of magical beliefs and their refutation by scientific physicians.
Until modern times this battle was not conclusively won. As
the sea ebbs and flows, so do scientific approaches sometimes
make encroachments upon the magical concept, and sometimes
recede before it—a pattern traced by Tempkin in his book *The
Falling Sickness*, to which all writers on the history of epilepsy
are indebted.

Hippocrates

The battle between the scientific and non-scientific attitude to

88

disease was first recorded in the book *On the Sacred Disease*, written by the physician Hippocrates in 400 BC. It was written for the layman and was an attack against popular superstition, magicians and charlatans who called the disease "sacred". Hippocrates said that the alleged divine character was only a cloak for ignorance and fraudulent practices. From the earliest times the greatest enemies of those with epilepsy have been superstition and fear, and as the approach of Hippocrates was scientific he represented a great advance. He rebutted the conception that epilepsy was caused by irrational forces and considered that it began in the brain. He said "the sacred disease appears to me to be no more divine nor more sacred than other diseases. . . . Men regard its nature and cause as divine from ignorance". In addition he considered it was often hereditary in origin.

The Comitial Disease

The "sacred disease" of the Greeks became not only the "morbus sacer" of the Romans but also the "morbus demonicus", a name used even by Martin Luther hundreds of years later. The belief that epilepsy was caused by an evil spirit probably led to practices like averting the evil eye by spitting on the patient; hence it was sometimes called "morbus insputatus". The Romans had yet another name, "morbus comitialis". It was explained by pseudo-Quintus Serenus, the poet-physician of the third century AD, that epilepsy prevented a true count of the vote, so that, if a person had a seizure in the Senate or Comitia, the meeting was suspended. Strangely, this idea is still known in Southern France, where Roman influence was strong. The epileptic was also regarded as unclean, so the sufferer was paradoxically labelled as having the "sacred disease" and yet never considered holy.

Galen

Galen, another physician of antiquity, lived some 500 years after Hippocrates, under the rule of the Roman empire. He believed that the ideal physician must be, in addition, a philosopher. Galen synthesised the Greek ideas of the four "elements", earth, air, fire and water with the notion of the four "humours" devised by Hippocrates, blood, phlegm, yellow bile and black bile. This scheme lasted into the seventeenth century, when it was discredited by Robert Boyle, though traces of such a view persist even in the twentieth century. Galen affirmed, like Hippocrates, that epileptic attacks started in the brain, and is often credited with the introduction into medical terminology of the word "aura". However, these warning signs of a fit were also described by Aretaeus of Cappodocia, who lived from AD 150 to 200. The word "aura", derived from the Latin, originally meant "a breeze". Galen recorded that a thirteen-year-old patient of his felt a sensation in his thigh which travelled up to his head, and another youth described a sensation "like a cold breeze".

St Valentine

In the Dark and early Middle Ages the popular desire to connect epilepsy with supernatural powers found a Christian counterpart in association with certain saints, especially St John in France and St Valentine in Germany. Apparently St Valentine acquired this honour simply because his name and the German word "*fallen*" sounded similar. Pilgrimages were undertaken to the Priory of St Valentine in Alsace, where, at the fifteenth century, a hospital for epileptics was built. There, patients underwent an elaborate ceremony with celebration of three Masses and a visit to the saint's grave. The view popular in the Middle Ages that epilepsy was contagious was held by both laymen and physicians alike. Since the breath was thought to be infectious, isolation hospitals were founded for epileptic patients. This view, though dropped in the sixteenth century, reappeared in another form in the eighteenth, when it was observed that the mere sight of epileptic sufferers could provoke seizures in the onlookers. Of course, now it was not the breath but, being the age of sensibility, the imagination!

Thomas Willis

While these discussions about supernatural powers were continuing, Thomas Willis was involved in studies of the anatomy and physiology of the brain. The illustrations to his anatomy books were drawn by no less a person than Sir Christopher Wren. Willis has been called the founder of "neurology" and in fact coined this term himself. He described fits in which the disturbance of consciousness was not so profound, as "universal convulsions". Those which were associated with periodic disorders of sensation would now be called temporal lobe epilepsy. At that time he was engaged in a study of the mind called psychology, and these mild epileptic disturbances he regarded as hysterical. This view persisted for 200 years down to the time of Charcot, when the hybrid concept "hystero-epilepsy" was invented.

Demoniacal possession

Most sixteenth- and seventeenth-century physicians were interested in demoniacal possession. Few doubted the existence of Satan, who was believed to be helped by a host of devils. It was discussed whether or not the devils and demons acted as a physical force, or whether their influence was restricted to the mind of man. Many physicians admitted that possession could occur, and their task was to distinguish it from epilepsy. This task was difficult enough, since possession frequently exhibited many characteristics of a fit. Jean Taxil, physician at Arles, thought that it was scarcely possible to find any case in the literature of one possessed with the devil who was not an epileptic, since in both conditions the sufferer fell in convulsions and frothed at the mouth.

The church was well aware of the close relation between epilepsy and possession, and F. M. Gnazzo's *Compendium Maleficarum* (Milan, 1608) describes the usual practice to determine whether a sick man was possessed—a distinction reviewed in an essay, "On the Demoniacs of the New Testament" by the eighteenth-century minister Hugh Farmer. The problem was further complicated by the theological necessity to investigate every case of "ecstatic rapture", to establish whether it was due to disease or divine power. The physicians were called in. They applied their irrational treatments of the "falling sickness" by enemas, purges, cuppings, fomentations, plasters and sweatings. If these treatments failed to give results, then it was presumed that a malign influence was at work.

The Age of Enlightenment

Before the Age of Enlightenment and the rejection of demoniacal possession, other irrational views appeared and disappeared, for example, that of the influence of the moon. Up to the end of the seventeenth century the influence of the moon upon epilepsy was taken as an established fact. In the late sixteenth century, Ferdinandus believed in one case that epilepsy had been caused by the patient spending a summer night under an olive tree "while the air was filled with a slight warmth from the light of the moon". Perhaps the lunar explanation of tides in Newtonian physics played its part, for even an enlightened physician like Richard Mead gave examples of epileptic attacks occurring regularly at certain phases of the moon. It is probably due to the authority of Mead that belief in the influence of the moon and other cosmic bodies survived so long in British medicine, even among men of such stature as John Hunter and Erasmus Darwin.

In France it was pointed out that the amount of heat the moon radiated was negligible, so that a mortal blow was dealt to the astrophysical theory of epilepsy. Tissot pointed out that, because epilepsy returned every month at the same day of the month, there was not necessarily a causal connection. His *Treatise on Epilepsy* (1770) was the first book on the subject to show all the characteristics of enlightenment in medicine. It was learned, scientific and readable. Tissot was to be found on the side of those opposing old beliefs for which no adequate reason could be found. Thus, not only did he reject the influence of the moon, but he also refused to accept the imagination of the pregnant mother as a cause of epilepsy. "Unfortunately, a change of mind which leads to the renunciation of old beliefs like demoniacal possession usually leads to the creation of new ones, and superstitions are often exchanged rather than abandoned."

The opinion prevailed that sexual excesses were harmful to epileptic people and yet complete continence might cause the disease. Later, the emphasis was on masturbation, which had been condemned on religious grounds. This superstition reached its zenith in the 1880s and at the annual meeting of the British Medical Association in 1880, a Dr Bacon reported that he had castrated two male epileptics, with the result that in one case there was a great improvement. Dr Hack Tuke asked under what condition such an operation would be indicated, and Dr Bacon replied, in cases of confirmed masturbation in incurable epileptic insanity. However, writing in 1881, Dr Gowers indicated that castration had proved unsuccessful as a treatment of epilepsy and said, "the possibility must not be overlooked, but the severe mental stress imposed by parents and educators upon the Onanist might sometimes lead to hysterical reactions".

In 1861 Sir Samuel Wilks published the first report on the treatment of epilepsy by bromides, though four years earlier Sir Charles Locock had discussed their use. Locock had first introduced it for "hysteria", but considered that the potassium in the potassium bromide he used was the effective element. In any event, this was the first effective treatment for epilepsy, though it was also observed that, when the treatment was discontinued, fits would recur, often with greater frequency. Sometimes, even, status epilepticus would occur (see below).

Treatments for epilepsy

The history of the treatment of epilepsy therefore shows, as with other diseases, a great variety of irrational manœuvres, some effective but most ineffective. Sir Edward Sieveking observed in 1858 that "there is not a substance in the *materia medica*, there is scarcely a substance in the world capable of passing through the gullet of man, that has not at one time or other enjoyed the reputation of being an anti-epileptic".

The medieval physician's régime of drugs, cauterisation and trephining followed ancient traditions. Of the surgical methods, cauterisation took first place. The hot iron was usually applied to several places on the head and sometimes to other regions, e.g. the shoulder-blades. The reason for this treatment was obscure. On the other hand, trephining, or making a small opening in the skull, was understandable, as a vent was made to allow the "mischievous matter" to escape. These were thought to be the cause of the trouble. However, the eighteenth-century physician Tissot saw trephining as a treatment for contusion of the skull. The history of the use of the trephine remained unbroken; it was only the reason for the operation that changed. It is interesting that Calvin Wells, in his book *Bones, Body and Disease*, notes that the use of slings as weapons and the trephine as a surgical instrument correspond geographically, an argument in favour of the practical rather than the animistic view of this device.

The change in therapeutics during the eighteenth century manifested itself by the rejection of a great many remedies that had been recommended by generations of physicians for their occult power over epilepsy. The enlightened eighteenth-century physicians could not allow the use of materials, such as human blood, bones and animal dung. However, the eighteenth-century physicians did not ignore therapeutics. Tissot recognised that the predisposing causes of epilepsy were not known, but that the patient should be kept on a healthy régime and free from excitement. The exact steps were decided for each individual. In short, this was a treatment of the epileptic patient rather than of epilepsy, which is still the key to the practice of good medicine.

Prevention

Suggestions for prevention of epilepsy can be studied in one of its most radical forms from the writings of Thomas Beddoes, a physician of the late eighteenth century. His "Essay on the Nature and Prevention of some of the Disorders, commonly called Nervous" explained that the disposition towards epilepsy was widespread. His work, however, leaves a frightening impression. Everybody suffering from the slightest nervous complaint might find himself threatened with future epilepsy and should therefore take steps to eradicate the disposition. The explanation of such exaggeration lies, perhaps, in the eighteenth century itself; the "enlightened" society which freed itself from the fear of witches and demons had surrendered to a new master, introspection, which led to hypochondria.

The view that epilepsy was infectious was a major error up to the beginning of the sixteenth century and still is not dead. It influenced treatment, which was not dissimilar to that given to lunatics and lepers, who also were isolated from the general population. The patients were often maltreated in chains, fetters and handcuffs. The humane pioneer Philippe Pinel freed the mental hospital patients at the end of the eighteenth century from their shackles, and conditions improved. However, as Dr Kathleen Jones points out, this humane policy was gradually reversed as the nineteenth century proceeded. By the end of it the wards of mental institutions again contained a great number of patients in locked wards under bad conditions. At present, in the case of both the mentally ill and the epileptic patients, the pendulum has swung once again to humane treatment, including treatment within the community itself. It is important to prevent the recurrence of the "sociological relapse" witnessed in the last century.

The later history of epilepsy

The history of epilepsy in the era of scientific medicine could be begun with Dr Richard Bright, a London physician born in the year of the French Revolution, 1789. He described a kidney disease with which his name is still associated and he noted also that an epileptic attack beginning in a small area of the outer surface of the brain or cortex was preceded by an aura. Dr

Bright was also notable as one of the first physicians to record the condition "status epilepticus". Though epilepsy had been known since antiquity, this particular condition, in which one fit rapidly follows another without consciousness being regained, had not been distinguished from any other. It was as recently as 1960 that Dr Richard Hunter wrote the history of status epilepticus. He indicated that, rather paradoxically, status epilepticus has been noted much more frequently since a really effective means of treatment had been discovered for epilepsy. The reason for this is still not clear.

Apart from clinical observation of the patient, other methods have also advanced the knowledge of epilepsy. Pathologists who examine the brain after the death of a patient have contributed. Walter Spielmeyer, born in Germany in 1879, was one such. His first thought was of a career in the church; however, he turned to medicine and worked with great energy, making important contributions on many diseases of the nervous system, particularly in pathology. He took small sections of the brain and studied them carefully under the microscope. He demonstrated that a shortage of blood in the brain could produce changes in the small and deeply placed part of the temporal lobe called "Ammon's horn". Later, others were to confirm that this area was responsible for the psychomotor seizures which occur in temporal lobe epilepsy.

Aleksei Yakovlevich Kozhevnikov was a distinguished Russian neurologist, born in 1836, who described an unusual type of seizure, starting in a small zone of the brain and remaining localised to that area for some minutes or even hours and resulting in prolonged attacks of twitching of a limb or face. This was a particularly noteworthy discovery, because quite often when an epileptic discharge starts, it spreads to involve the whole brain. A prolonged limited attack of epilepsy is sometimes given the name of its discoverer, but more often the long Latin title, *epilepsia partialis continua*, is used.

Charles Edward Brown-Séquard, born in 1817 on the small island of Mauritius in the Indian Ocean, travelled widely in Europe and the United States, and was among the earliest to realise the value of animal experiments in medicine. He began to study guinea pigs who developed epileptic seizures following electrical stimulation. This type of experiment continues today, not only in the study of epilepsy but also in other branches of medicine. Brown-Séquard remained interested in epilepsy for much of his life and was one of the first people to prescribe bromide in the convulsive disorders, the only really effective medicine at that time.

Jean Martin Charcot was one of a number of distinguished French neurologists who practised in the middle and latter part of the nineteenth century. Born in Paris in 1825, most of his career centred around the hospital of La Salpetrière in Paris. He joined battle not only with Hughlings Jackson, an English neurologist who will be described later, but also with Brown-Séquard. The arguments covered a particular type of attack now known as Jacksonian epilepsy. However, Charcot is perhaps best known for his work on hysteria. Hysterical attacks at that time were very common and mimicked convulsions. His fame was such that doctors from all over Europe visited him at the Salpetrière Hospital. One of these was Sigmund Freud, who was at that time unknown; he watched Charcot's clinical demonstrations of patients with neurological disorders, and the use of hypnosis in treatment. Later Freud wrote about the association of epilepsy and hysteria and the use of hypnosis in psychiatric treatment. Freud also published a study of Dostoievski, the famous Russian novelist who suffered from epilepsy (see chapter XII).

Britain has provided two important figures in the history of epilepsy. Sir William Gowers lived from 1845 to 1915 and worked in London, particularly at the National Hospital in Queen Square. His main interest was in the clinical aspects of epilepsy, and he wrote a book still widely read, *The Borderlands of Epilepsy*. In this are described conditions other than epilepsy which occur spasmodically, for example, migraine. Gowers was a passionate man who had a great interest in shorthand, which he felt was essential to success in life. The story goes that he stopped his carriage in a busy London street and alighted in order to persuade a young man who was passing by of the value of acquiring knowledge of shorthand!

Perhaps the most important contributor to the neurology of epilepsy was Dr Hughlings Jackson. He was born in 1835 and was a contemporary of Gowers. Like Brown-Séquard and Gowers, he too worked at the National Hospital. His name is attached to one type of fit now widely known as Jacksonian epilepsy. This is no accident, for his cousin-wife had just such attacks. He noted that, if the fit started in the toe, a tight band around it could prevent the epileptic movements spreading up the leg and later involving the whole body. However, more important than the exact description of one type of rare attack was his formation of the concept of epilepsy, which has stood the test of time and, in particular, has been confirmed by EEG studies fifty years later. He defined epilepsy as "an occasional, sudden, massive, rapid and local discharge of the grey matter". He further divided the brain into higher and lower levels with corresponding higher and lower functions. He wrote copiously on epilepsy and other neurological subjects, and Dr William Lennox, himself a great American epileptologist, says in his history of epilepsy that Jackson "opened the door of hope to this hitherto hopeless disease".

As already mentioned, the treatment of epilepsy with an effective drug, bromide, began in the late nineteenth century, even though the rationale for this method was quite inaccurate. The next stage was the introduction by Dr Alfred Hauptmann from Germany of the barbiturate drugs. In 1912 he published the first paper on the use of luminal, now called phenobarbitone; the beginning of a safe and really effective treatment for epilepsy. Not until 1939, when Drs Merritt and Putnam in the United States introduced phenytoin did the next really efficacious drug become available, to be followed by troxidone in 1946, described by Drs Richards and Perlstein. This again was a real advance, because it was the first effective drug in the treatment of *petit mal* epilepsy.

In more recent times contributions to the story of epilepsy have been made from America. The Drs Gibbs, husband and wife team, have made great contributions in the field of electro-encephalography, and Dr William Lennox not only devoted much of his life to the study of epilepsy, but wrote a two-volume work embracing the current knowledge of this disease. This book, *Epilepsy and Related Disorders*, has historical references and numerous case studies of his own patients. The list should be lengthened to include Dr Wilder Penfield, who worked at the Montreal Neurological Institute on the treatment of epilepsy by surgical operation. By skilful observation during operations he has, in addition, increased understanding of the basic mechanisms of the brain function. However, in spite of extensive research, a vast number of unsolved problems of causation and treatment remain, and the story of epilepsy is still far from complete.

CHAPTER ELEVEN

Some historical epileptic people

WHAT DO the following people have in common—the apostle Paul, Buddha, Alexander the Great, Julius Caesar, Mohamed and Pascal, Flaubert, Paganini, Byron, Napoleon, Swinburne, Van Gogh, Pope Pius IX? These and other famous people are said to have suffered from epilepsy. Whether they did in fact is difficult to determine. Quite often the evidence on which the diagnosis rests consists only of tantalising fragments seen through unscientific eyes. Nevertheless the lives of three of these famous people will be mentioned briefly in an attempt to determine the truth of such a diagnosis, and most of all to indicate that there have been eccentric people with epilepsy, as well as happy and unhappy people with epilepsy. The truth emerges that most people with epilepsy are neither brilliant nor moody but unexceptional and of unremarkable temperament.

Julius Caesar

Julius Caesar was a baffling, contradictory and glamorous character. He has been regarded as the greatest of the Romans, and was apparently of sound health apart from having night-mares. However, during his numerous campaigns, on two occasions he apparently had epileptic fits. In spite of this he built a vast empire and clearly the "falling sickness" was no limitation.

St Paul

According to tradition Saul of Tarsus suffered from fits. The facts are scanty, but in the ninth chapter of the Acts of the Apostles it is learnt that he was proceeding to Damascus to persecute a new sect—the Christians. On the way he fell to the ground, hearing a voice saying, "Saul, Saul, why persecutest thou me." For three days after that he was without sight, and neither ate nor drank. This can hardly be considered evidence for a diagnosis of epilepsy, but it must be taken in conjunction with the words he wrote in his second letter to the Corinthians, chapter XII, where the famous passage containing the words "a thorn in the flesh" occurs. "For this thing, I besought the Lord thrice that it might depart from me. . . . I take pleasure in infirmities, in reproaches, in necessities, in persecutions, in distresses for Christ's sake, for when I am weak, then I am strong."

Whatever St Paul's infirmity was, he did not consider it incapacitating. Was the "thorn in the flesh" epilepsy? Fresh evidence is unlikely to come to light now, though there are other views as to its nature. William Lennox suggested an "emotional reaction to the voice of Conscience in combination with migraine". Indeed, Tertullian as early as the second century had suggested the diagnosis of "recurrent headaches".

Rudyard Kipling suggested that Paul suffered from a "deadly Syrian malaria, which strikes like a snake", accounting for the collapse on the road to Damascus. Whether St Paul had epilepsy or not remains enigmatic.

Vincent van Gogh

The career, the illness and the death of Vincent van Gogh have interested many medical writers; in spite of the fact that he lived so recently medical records are scanty, and there has been great controversy about his condition. Schizophrenia, psychopathic personality and epilepsy have all been suggested.

Vincent van Gogh was born in 1853 at Groot Zundert, where his father was a pastor. His early adult life was as a Methodist minister and, in spite of privation and family disputes there was no sign of epilepsy. However, he did have considerable swings of mood from depression to elation.

After his father's death in 1885 he went to Paris, where he lived with his brother Theo. There he stayed for two years in the circle of Toulouse-Lautrec and Gauguin. It was in Paris that he started to drink absinthe, and in the winter of 1887 he first had convulsions.

In the autumn of 1888 he invited Gauguin to join him in Arles, where together they drank heavily and visited brothels. On Christmas Eve van Gogh quarrelled with Gauguin, and after this cut off part of his own ear, which was then delivered in a parcel to a prostitute, who gave it to the proprietress, who in her turn gave it to the police. This bizarre behaviour occurred while van Gogh was in a delirious state and he was admitted to hospital.

Dr Felix Rey attended van Gogh when he was first admitted and considered that he was suffering from a form of epilepsy with hallucinations, episodes of agitation and confusion provoked by drinking absinthe to excess. No other clinical diagnosis was made. Alcohol was withheld and van Gogh was given large doses of bromide. However, it seems in addition to alcoholism he suffered from severe swings of mood, according to his letters to his brother Theo. This was supported by Dr Rey's observation that Van Gogh had a great urge to paint after recovery from periods of despair.

Absinthe drinking was known to have bad effects even at that time, so much so that by 1914 its sale was prohibited altogether. The particular constituent at fault was probably the volatile oil thujone, known to cause states of agitation with hallucinations. Van Gogh took large quantities of absinthe, when he was allowed to go into Arles from hospital, and following this fits always occurred. These fits were controlled when he was in hospital off alcohol and taking the bromide prescribed. It therefore seems unlikely that van Gogh suffered from temporal lobe epilepsy as has been suggested, rather that he had absinthe poisoning, with convulsions as a result. To use current terminology, van Gogh probably suffered from non-focal symptomatic epilepsy.

Modern epileptic case histories

Finally here are brief sketches of two epileptics who are still alive. These people have met with success despite their affliction. The first was serving in the American forces during the war in Okinawa when he first developed epilepsy. He was discharged from the navy, and was told that he had a brain wave disturbance and would have to take medication. In spite of this he gained a scholarship to an art institute, but had great difficulty in finding a job after the four-year course. The question: "Have you any physical disability?" was always asked by the employer, and when the honest answer was "Yes", the response was "Sorry, but . . ."

Once, after successfully obtaining a job, this artist-in-the-making arrived nervously at the studio and almost at once had a fit, which landed him in hospital without a job. After this attack he managed to continue with free-lance work and gradually his morale improved. He became engaged, but attacks recurred and once more a spell in hospital was necessary. There he met an older man who had epilepsy but was married with a family and held a steady job. The sharing of experiences with his fellow sufferer helped both of them to face life again with greater serenity. His engagement was dissolved by mutual consent, and visits to studios and art agencies recommenced with the usual rebuffs. Gradually, however, his skill increased and the demand for his work likewise. Still on anti-convulsant tablets he has become a successful artist in the commercial field, has had shows at many galleries, and his pictures have been sold all over the United States.

The second story is also from America and concerns a young

television actress who continues to perform in front of the cameras, run a home and look after a family in spite of attacks. "I have come to terms with my illness," she said, "I've decided not to retreat from life or to become a recluse." This illness struck the patient in her eighth month of pregnancy while in a doctor's waiting-room. In spite of an attack at that stage of pregnancy, her child born the next day was quite healthy. Her second fit occurred in front of a studio audience while she was a panellist on a TV show. In spite of fits she continues at work; she regards epilepsy as inconvenient because of its surprise element, but consoles herself that there is no pain. This plucky actress is able to lead a full life despite epilepsy. Her reaction to this handicap is not unusual in those with epilepsy.

CHAPTER TWELVE

Epilepsy in literature

EPILEPSY HAS been of interest to non-medical writers from earliest to modern times. A. E. Housman, poet and classical scholar, wrote in his poem "Oracles":

> "Oh Priestess, what you cry is clear, and sounds good sense, I think it,
> But let the screaming echoes out and froth your mouth no more."

He therefore suggested that, in early Greek times, the priestess at the Cave of Oracles simulated an epileptic fit when she was consulted. A more detailed description of an epileptic fit, given by Lucretius in *De Rerum Natura*, was quoted in on page 5.

It is obvious that Lucretius had observed fits, and the same is true in the account in the New Testament from St Luke, chapter IX.

> "Master, I beseech thee, look upon my son; for he is mine only child: and lo, a spirit taketh him, and he suddenly crieth out; and it teareth him that he foameth again and, bruising him, hardly departeth from him."

Another version of the biblical story in St Mark, chapter IX, is also worth mentioning because of the last verse. In this, Jesus comments on the "foul spirit" responsible for the epileptic attack as follows: "This kind come forth by nothing but by prayer and fasting." The interest is in the reference to fasting, because this indeed has formed the basis of a twentieth-century treatment of epilepsy. The patient first fasts for a few days, then is introduced to a special diet. However, with the increase in the number and variety of anti-convulsant medications, this therapy is at present rarely used.

The words "devil" and "unclean spirit" are used in these biblical passages as an explanation of the affliction, and Origen, one of the early Christian fathers, writing in AD 254, admitted that the boy was suffering from epilepsy, adding: "Physicians may offer natural theories since, according to their view, it is not an unclean spirit, but a bodily affliction which presents itself." Thus even in ancient times there was a marked difference in opinion about the cause of fits.

This is borne out in the account of Apuleius, a contemporary of Galen, who writes as follows: "The spinning of the potter's wheel will easily infect a man suffering from this disease [epilepsy] with its own giddiness; for the sight of its rotations weakens his already feeble mind, and the potter is more effective than the magician for casting epileptics into convulsions." However, of particular interest is the precipitation of fits. It is presumed to be not so much from the rotation of the wheel itself as from the flashing of the reflected light from the wheel as it turned rapidly. Nowadays, television sets rather than potters' wheels may induce fits in this way!

Epilepsy in Shakespeare

The works of Shakespeare contain a few references to epilepsy. Kent, Lear's faithful servant, when in extreme anger with Oswald, says, "A plague upon your epileptic visage." Perhaps this is a reflection of a common Elizabethan attitude not only to epilepsy but also to invective. Of Othello, Shakespeare wrote that he was goaded beyond endurance by Iago. Cassio discovers him unconscious with Iago standing beside him.

Cassio: "What's the matter?"
Iago: "My lord is fallen into an epilepsy. This is his second fit;
he had one yesterday."
Cassio: "Rub him about the temples."
Iago: "No, forbear;
The lethargy must have his quiet course:
If not, he foams at mouth and by and by,
Breaks out to savage madness."

Of course, Cassio was extremely credulous and Iago was a liar,
but it does seem that Othello was so overwrought that he was
overtaken by what an Elizabethan audience would have called
epilepsy.

One last example, and the most interesting, comes from
Julius Caesar. Casca gives an eye-witness account of how Mark
Antony offered Caesar a crown three times, and each time
Caesar rejected it, then, "he swounded". Casca continues:

"He fell down in the market place and foamed at the mouth
and was speechless."
Brutus: "'Tis very like he hath the falling sickness."
Cassius: "No, Caesar hath it not, but you and I, honest Casca,
we have the falling sickness."

Dostoevski

Dostoevski's works contain the most comprehensive account of
various forms of epilepsy, and they show something of his own
affliction as well as how it could be turned to literary use.
Epilepsy figures in *The Idiot*, where Prince Myshkin suffered
from it; similarly, Smirdyakov in *The Brothers Karamazov*,
Kirilov in *The Possessed* and Nellie in *The Insulted and Injured*. In
The Idiot epilepsy plays the most important part, and the attacks
of Prince Myshkin are usually regarded as similar to those of
Dostoevski himself, in particular the feeling of increased vitality
that preceded the attacks: ". . . all his emotions, all his doubts,
all his anxiety calmed together to be changed in a sovereign
serenity made up of lighted joy, harmony and hope; then his

reason was raised up to the understanding of the final cause". However, this feeling was not the only aspect of the Prince's fits, for he apparently recalled the very beginning of his attack in which a cry "burst from his chest". This latter is almost certainly author's licence, for most people have little knowledge of even earlier parts of a fit than this. In *The Possessed* again the feeling of serenity is mentioned; Kirilov says, "There are some instants, they last five or six seconds, when you suddenly feel the presence of the eternal harmony, then you have reached it . . . it is a clear, indisputable, absolute feeling. You suddenly embrace the entire creation and you say, well, it is like that, it is true."

A note from the diary of Dostoevski reveals other aspects of his attacks which would nowadays be labelled temporal lobe epilepsy. "This morning, at 8.45, interruption of my thoughts, transported into other years, dreams, dreamy states, dreaminess . . . guilt." So the transcendental feeling of many of his attacks was by no means universal, and this is certainly true of most who suffer from fits. Other aspects are well described by Margiad Evans, an authoress who later died of a brain tumour.

Margiad Evans

Her autobiography, *A Ray of Darkness*, is remarkable. Somewhere W. B. Yeats writes the line, "beauty that we have won from bitterest hours", and this line fairly sums up the haunting quality of the book. Perhaps it is too long, and does not entirely succeed in transmuting experience into a work of art, but her bravery and stoic acceptance of a personal catastrophe must be saluted.

Margiad's description of her first fit is quoted in chapter I (pp. 6–7). After her second epileptic fit she writes, "I had never really thought until then that I myself was going to die soon, but now I did. I cannot think why, for I was perfectly well aware that people do not die of fits."

Another autobiographical account of a brain tumour and

attacks occurs in *Journeys around my Skull*, by Frigyes Karinthy, who died after completing the account.

Anthony Chuzzlewit

Charles Dickens describes epileptic attacks which lead to death in the aged Anthony Chuzzlewit. "He had fallen from his chair in a fit and lay there gasping for breath." The surgeon was hastily called, but in spite of bleeding and other remedies the fits apparently continued. Next morning the old man was gabbling in a strange tongue, and when he was wheeled to the window he expired. Jonas, who had earlier laced his father's cough medicine with poison, considered that he was responsible for the death. His father, however, had discerned that something was amiss with the medicine and only pretended to drink it. No one knows what poison Dickens had in mind to cause convulsions, but strychnine would have been appropriate, as Sir Russell Brain observed in his essay on "Dickensian Diagnoses", one of a collection entitled *Some Reflections on Genius*. He further commented that old Anthony appeared to have died of a series of convulsions due to cerebral arteriosclerosis common in old age. Using modern terminology Anthony Chuzzlewit suffered from symptomatic epilepsy.

This does not exhaust the accounts of epilepsy in literature. Even Samuel Taylor Coleridge wrote of it in the poem *The Ancient Mariner*:

> "I moved my lips—the Pilot shrieked
> and fell down in a fit."

Faints are also important, for example in George Farquhar's play, *The Beaux' Stratagem*. It is possible even to postulate that George Eliot's character Silas Marner suffered from some form of temporal lobe attacks, as his behaviour was marked by circumscribed periods of amnesia.

CHAPTER THIRTEEN

Epilepsy and crime

In the past it has been suggested that many crimes are committed by epileptic people perhaps during or just after a fit, and this view is still current at the present time. It has also been suggested that epileptic sufferers show a predilection to violence and sexual assault. However, a forensic psychiatrist, Peter Scott, wrote in an article on the medical aspects of delinquency that "epileptics are not particularly prone to crime, and when they do commit a crime they do not (despite the older textbooks) show any particular predilection for murder, rape or arson". He continued, "most very destructive or aggressive offences, including arson and murder, are not committed by epileptics".

Juul-Jensen found, in a Danish department of neurology, that the frequency of crime among men with epilepsy was 9·5 per cent, identical to the figure for the general population. He also observed that female epileptics have a crime rate of 1·5 per cent, which is similar to that of women without epilepsy. In addition, Juul-Jensen found no particular correlation between seizures and criminal acts and again, like Peter Scott, no preponderance of arson, sexual or violent crimes. Kurt Alström of Sweden, in a study of the penal records of 345 adult male epileptic patients, found no acts of homicide over a ten-year period, though he did find a slight excess of crimes in the epileptic group compared with a group of non-epileptics. However, all the crimes were of a minor nature. It appeared that neither crimes of violence towards others nor crime occurring during the seizure were encountered. Hill and Pond indicate from their experience of epileptic patients, both in and out of hospital, that dangerous or violent behaviour occurring during or immediately after an epileptic fit was rarely observed.

Levin examined a series of patients admitted to the Boston Psychopathic Hospital, in a "clouded mental state as a result of an epileptic attack". He observed that, though these patients were confused and potentially aggressive, they were quite unable to carry out aggressive acts because these usually require planning and integrated behaviour.

On the subject of violent crime, Fenton and Unwin published an interesting study of a man who became depressed and in the small hours of the morning killed his wife; he subsequently attacked his daughter, and then threw himself from a window. He fell thirteen feet on to his head and fractured his skull. Some two years later he was observed to fall unconscious to the ground, though no convulsive movements were noticed. He continued to have similar occasional attacks and, on subsequent investigation, a temporal lobe focus was discovered. It turned out on further questioning that he had had very brief attacks on the day before his crime, and even before that he had ear disease which had spread to affect the mastoid bone, behind the ear. It is known from the study of other patients that such infections may spread to the brain with little outside evidence of this.

Doctors who examined the patient concluded that his epilepsy had been one of the factors which had precipitated his depressive illness. In fact, the association of depressive illness and murder is not infrequently reported. It characteristically occurs in the early morning, and the murder of relatives is followed by attempted or successful suicide. There was no evidence that the murder itself had been carried out during an automatism.

The Ruby trial

The assassination of President Kennedy on 22nd November 1963 and the shooting by Jack Ruby two days later of his supposed assassin, Lee Harvey Oswald, is still a clear memory for many people. It is examined here for the following reasons: first, because some aspects indicate the difficulties in the diagnosis of epilepsy, and secondly it raises the questions about epileptic automatisms which are of interest. A final question concerns the possibility of performing criminal acts during epileptic fits.

At the trial of Jack Ruby it was suggested by his defence lawyer that Ruby suffered from epilepsy and murdered Oswald in a state of epileptic automatism. The verbatim account of the trial shows how many disagreements there are about epilepsy and related matters between experts, be they physicians, psychiatrists or electro-encephalographers. In the course of life Ruby had had a number of head injuries such as have been known to lead to epilepsy; but he had had no convulsive attacks, though he had suffered from brief spells, lasting perhaps half a minute, associated with feelings of uneasiness. In these he felt alone and that he might "black-out", though he never actually did. These spells occurred perhaps once a month. It was also noted that no one in Ruby's family suffered from epilepsy.

The next part of the evidence centred round the EEG. The "brain tracing" was mostly normal apart from a few short runs in which there was an unusual feature, a pattern of theta waves (see chapter IV) over the temporal area which may be seen when the patient is slightly drowsy and has been called "psychomotor variant" by the well-known electro-encephalographer Dr Gibbs. But no definite epileptic waves were observed, so there was little evidence for a diagnosis of epilepsy.

As for the further suggestion that the killing was done in a state of automatism following an epileptic fit, an examination of the events may help to elucidate this. Ruby walked into the basement of the police station, pushed through the crowd, taking out his revolver as he went. He faced Oswald and said, "You killed the President, you rat." He fired one shot and was then arrested by the policemen who had let him through. Later he professed in court that his memory was hazy for all these events, but there was no definite loss of memory.

An epileptic automatism would certainly have been quite different. Professor H. Gastaut stated that Ruby would have hurled himself forward through the crowds, fumbling in his pockets for a gun. He would have fired the gun repeatedly and clumsily. After the incident Ruby would have been found to be confused, unable to speak coherently, or know where he was. It would have appeared like a combination of mild drunkenness and absent-mindedness. The difference between this and what actually did happen is clear. Ruby almost certainly did not suffer from epilepsy, and automatism is even more unlikely.

Why Ruby killed, or what was the psychological basis of his action, will probably never be known. It is unfortunate that his crime became linked in this way with epilepsy. Naturally, those concerned with epileptic patients strongly objected. The court-house was picketed by members of the National Epilepsy League, and in the *Journal of the American Association* of 13 April 1964, appeared a letter signed by five experts on epilepsy and electro-encephalography. This letter stated that "neither the clinical history nor the electro-encephalograph of Mr Ruby indicated definite evidence of epilepsy". These doctors then affirmed that "epilepsy is not associated with acts of violence" and that "epileptics are as safe to be with as any other group, except in extremely rare and usually predictable situations". There was discussion as to whether the American Medical Association should make a similar affirmation about the occurrence of violent behaviour in epileptic patients. It was decided, however, that such a statement might in itself lead to more adverse publicity, so no affirmation was made.

What is the experience of other experts in epilepsy on the matter of crime committed during fits? W. Lennox in the United States encountered two murders by epileptic patients in thirty-five years and in neither was there evidence that it was performed during an epileptic attack. Professor Gastaut had, in the course of twenty years' study in France, encountered only three criminal acts among epileptic people. These had no serious medico-legal implications and there was no evidence in any of these of automatism. Wilder Penfield, who pioneered temporal lobe surgery, noted that acts of violence were almost unknown in the whole literature of epilepsy. These views are confirmed in a recent study of crime during automatisms by Gunn and Fenton, who examined epileptic criminals in Broadmoor Hospital and elsewhere. They came to the conclusion that violent acts in a close time relationship to epileptic fits were rare. However, they have found that the prevalence of epilepsy (7–8 per thousand men) in prisons and borstal was significantly higher than in the general population and they are unable to give an explanation for it. This is yet another of the question marks that surround the subject of epilepsy and further research is obviously required.

In conclusion, there seems no real evidence that criminal acts are common in epileptic patients either between or during fits.

CHAPTER FOURTEEN

The care of the epileptic person

APART FROM doctors and nurses, many different groups of people may be concerned with the epileptic person, for example, teachers, employers, local government authorities, social workers, even insurance brokers. Let us consider their dealings with the epileptic.

Schooling of the child with fits

The education of the epileptic child poses many problems. First of all, fits may interfere with schooling. If major fits occur in the classroom say once a week, the disturbance will be such that it will be difficult for the patient to remain in the ordinary class of a normal school. This is extremely unfortunate, because the epileptic child may then have to be separated from children of his own age and be educated in a special setting. He may already feel, even at this young age, that he is different because of his attacks, and a psychological difficulty may be created and fostered. This feeling of separation and inferiority may pursue an epileptic child for the rest of his life.

If education is neglected he will be less ready for a job and a new vicious circle of employment difficulty and the psychological problems engendered therefrom will arise.

However, the situation may not be as gloomy as this if attacks of this major kind occur regularly when the child is in bed at home; then there is no reason why he should not be able to attend a normal school. Other types of attack may occur in the classroom and perhaps not even the teacher, unless she was warned, would realise that they had taken place. A *petit mal* attack can pass almost unnoticed and the child is well able to cope with his lessons. However, even though these attacks are brief, they may still interfere with the memory. If the attacks are very frequent this may lead to a poorer performance by the child than expected from his intelligence scores; this fact sometimes leads to the discovery of *petit mal*—as a result of the child's poor performance he is observed more closely and attacks are noticed. However, when the diagnosis of *petit mal* epilepsy has been made and medication started, the child's scholastic performance will usually improve.

The aim of parents and teachers is to keep all children, if possible, in the ordinary school. Dr T. K. Whitmore, of the Department of Education, says that this is possible for 96 out of 100 epileptic children. It is important to tell the teacher about the child's problem and reduce the teacher's anxieties. Often worry on the part of the teacher that the child may have an attack in class leads to tension, which may, in turn, be transmitted to the child so that the situation gets steadily worse.

Sometimes it is even a good thing that the other children should be told that one of their fellows has this disability. Clearly this step has to be taken with caution, because the young are notorious in their ability to tease and persecute a fellow who has a disability. It may be wise, however, to leave the other children in the class in ignorance, particularly as parents of children, not the teacher or the children themselves, are often the ones who complain about the epileptic child. For this reason the headmaster of a smart private school may not be sympathetic towards the epileptic child because he fears repercussions from the parents of other children.

Even if ordinary classes are impossible for the epileptic child, special classes in ordinary schools are better than the special school itself, although the advantages of the school for epileptic children must not be forgotten in some special instances. There, the children may receive just the extra educational help they require and, in addition, special doctors look after them. In England, Lingfield Hospital School caters for children with fits. However, in a recent survey it was discovered that the children who attended this had relatively infrequent fits and were there because of other behavioural difficulties or because of poor social circumstances. Lingfield School is valuable because, in the final years, instead of academic subjects, more practical subjects are taught, and in this way the child can be gently weaned from school into training and then to suitable employment.

If the child is mentally retarded and has fits in addition, a special school will be required. However, there is no reason why such children should not be taught simple tasks and trained to carry out repetitive work so as to obtain employment, sometimes commercially, though more often in a protected workshop.

Teachers must be persuaded, like parents, not to be over-protective towards the epileptic child. It is important that they are not unduly lenient; the handicapped should never be singled out for special favours or, for that matter, special punishments. There are relatively few features of school life into which the epileptic child should not be permitted to enter. The restriction applies to certain forms of physical recreation; rope climbing is one example, and swimming another unless there is close supervision. When fits are frequent and out of control, these should not be permitted.

The performance of certain epileptic children in school may be well above average, and a college or university place should be found for them. This is not always easy because of resistance on the part of the authorities.

There is nothing to preclude the epileptic patient from almost any vocation of his choice. There is no doubt that he will encounter difficulties, but it is probably better that he undertakes something which he fervently desires than that he be fobbed off with a second-best occupation.

There are two main groups of patients who have difficulty. An example of the first would be a man in his late 20s or 30s. He has already had training and a satisfactory work record before developing fits. Characteristic of the second group is the teenager whose fits began in childhood and who has never had a job, so has neither training nor experience. Without work both of these will lie about at home, getting in the way of the wife or mother as she looks after the house. They are bored, they lose all self-respect; in such a situation fits may become more frequent. Eventually the patient no longer wants to go out looking for work, and even if he does his pessimistic attitude is not likely to endear him to a would-be employer.

Like many perfectly normal teenagers the boy or girl with epilepsy who has just left school may not be clear about what type of work he would like, but he has the added difficulty of his condition. He may drift, like them, from one employer to another, but in his case not all the changes will be voluntary and he has less freedom to try jobs out. He may long to become a motor mechanic, but he is not allowed to drive a car because of his attacks so that ambition is killed. He loses heart after this and similar rebuffs, and may finally turn delinquent, more out of boredom than positive intent.

The main duty of a doctor in dealing with either of these groups of patients is to see that their epileptic fits are well controlled and decide whether surgical treatment is indicated or not. Apart from his medical role the doctor can help the patient greatly in other ways. Frank discussion of his capabilities is essential not only with regard to the attacks, but also with consideration of his intelligence and background. The doctor can, from his experience of other patients, suggest suitable outlets. The type and frequency of attack is of great importance. Occasional nocturnal fits are hardly a barrier to any type of position. The doctor too may be aware of various governmental and voluntary agents that can help the patient. The patient can be put in touch with these by a suitable letter or phone call.

The wife or parent needs reassurance concerning the diagnosis and the treatment of epilepsy. When all investigations have been undertaken and the patient is taking anti-convulsant drugs, relatives will feel less anxious and will then be of great help to the patient. A secure home without tension is an extremely good base from which the patient can venture to look for employment. After helping the relatives in this way there is a further important duty for the doctor. At the patient's request he may send a report to a would-be employer. Such a report would indicate that the patient was under treatment, that the work in question was suitable, and that in the event of any difficulties the doctor would be prepared to help. Such a method aids the employer and makes the first few days in a new job much easier for the patient.

Problems with jobs

How many patients with epilepsy do in fact have employment difficulties? In a survey of epilepsy in fourteen general practices in England by Pond, 64 out of 157 patients with epilepsy who were of employable age had job problems. A similar proportion was discovered by Porter in another survey. Out of 100 patients seen at the Central Middlesex Hospital, 34 had employment difficulties. Some of these problems were caused by the fits themselves, others were the result of the employer's attitude. This was well summed up in an article during 1961 in the *Journal of the American Medical Association* in which attention was drawn not only to the *capacity* of the epileptic patient for work, but also of his *acceptability* for work. The employer has a resistance to employing a patient subject to fits, partly based on an irrational fear of epilepsy from the past but, in addition, because of a concern with more up-to-date problems such as insurance against industrial accidents. Many employers feel that epileptic patients are particularly liable to accidents and therefore a great risk, and that they are more likely to take time off work. Other ideas often expressed are that stress may bring on the attacks, that epileptic patients are not physically capable of work, and that they are of unsound mind. These views on the employment of epileptic patients will now be considered in more detail.

In a survey conducted by the U.S. Department of Labor, comparison was made between the performance of epileptic and non-epileptic subjects. Results showed that attendance rates were equally good in the two groups and that, though there was a slightly higher accident rate in the group of epileptic patients, the "time-lost rate" was actually lower for them than for the non-epileptic group. The figures were per 100 scheduled work days, 0·02 days lost for the epileptic as compared with 0·13 for the other group. Similar findings have been noted by the U.S. Veterans Administration Hospitals and by other doctors and agencies both in the U.S.A. and in Europe. It may seem surprising that the accident rate is not much higher in the epileptic group. We can only assume that the employed epileptic person is aware that he has a disability which may increase his liability to accidents and he is careful that accidents unrelated to the fits are kept to a minimum. No doubt he realises the difficulty of getting employment and makes sure that his absentee rate and time-keeping are at least as good, if not better, than his unimpaired colleagues.

The employer may fear that stress will increase attacks; in fact, the experience of many doctors and others is that the reverse is true. Alertness needed at work inhibits the occurrence of fits, and suitable employment is often a valuable step in achieving good control of fits. Idleness and sleep are the worst enemies of good fit control. It was observed during the bombing in World War II that there was no increase in the number of epileptic attacks recorded in epileptic colonies in either the United Kingdom or Europe.

The question of the epileptic patient not being intellectually or psychologically up to the standard of his fellow workers has already been shown to be untrue elsewhere in this book and will not be discussed again—see pp. 83–7.

Another difficulty often raised by employers is that other employees will be upset by witnessing fits. It is true that no one likes seeing a fit. However, in time this fear can be overcome by educating the public through media such as newspapers and television. Knowledge can help to dispel this fear, and in fact many workers become adept at aiding their less fortunate colleagues in the event of an attack at work.

Workers' compensation

The difficulty of workers' compensation is a very real one. At least in the United States it has been partially solved, but the final solution is still awaited. Such unsatisfactory suggestions as voluntary waiving of the epileptics' rights to compensation are clearly unsatisfactory. A more amicable system is called the "second injury fund". This fund is raised from taxes, and is used in the event of a disabled person having a second accident. In this way the employer of a handicapped patient is able to share any financial burden with a much wider group. Barrow and Fabing in their book *Epilepsy and the Law* have reviewed all such difficulties in detail and have stimulated interest in this topic and others concerned with integration of the epileptic patient into the general community.

Many government organisations and official bodies in general will not employ epileptic patients—the Police Force, Armed Services, and some religious bodies, including the Catholic Church, are examples. Sometimes if an employee does develop epilepsy while in one of these agencies, he is retained rather than forced to retire. However, the United States Civil Service Commission, one of the largest employers in that country, put forward quite different views in 1958. In their pamphlet *Employment of Epileptics in the Federal Service*, they positively approved of the employment of patients with well controlled fits in certain posts. It appears that a minor victory has been won but, as will be seen from the succeeding paragraph, much remains to be done. The hearts of many employers are still hardened against the epileptic worker.

Again in the United States a survey of *The Attitudes of the Employer to Workers Compensation Insurance Cycle and the Rehabilitation Process* was carried out by Dr Frank Risch. He used a questionnaire to collect information from 500 companies in Arizona employing 64,000 people, of whom less than 0·1 per cent were epileptics. This compares with the occurrence of epilepsy in the general population of about 1 in every 100–300 persons; hence there are fewer epileptics in employment than there should be. In fact, only 12 of the total number of 314 firms who replied had epileptics in their premises and in addition, only 12 reported that they had no restrictions in employing epileptics. Three-fourths of the companies said that they would not knowingly hire an epileptic worker and nearly a quarter of the companies stated that they would sack such a worker if he was discovered to have a fit at work. More propaganda is still needed on behalf of epileptic workers.

Secrecy, as William Lennox stated, is the bugbear of epilepsy. The patient should be able to tell the employer that he has fits, but so many patients get no nearer a job than making a confession to a would-be employer that they suffer from fits; hence, many patients suppress the truth and this may account for the small percentage of employers discovered in the survey of Dr Risch. Every doctor who deals with epileptic patients knows that they often obtain employment without telling the employer of their fits. If there is a danger in such deceit, then the patient will usually be told gently and firmly that such a lie is unwise; however, there a doctor's duty must rest, but there are other fields of activity that the doctor can pursue.

Epihab

In 1956 Dr Frank Risch began in Los Angeles an unusual experiment. He founded an industrial firm under the odd name of Epihab, standing for epilepsy rehabilitation. The idea was to employ epileptics, train them and in the end place them in ordinary businesses or industrial work. There are now several similar factories flourishing in parts of the United States. Not only have the problems of production been solved but also some of those connected with compensation. The epileptic worker there uses hand tools and electrical equipment, and in addition power tools such as hand saws which have in the past been regarded as extremely dangerous for the epileptic. In the first four years of operation, 1956–60, accidents resulted in the loss of only one hour for every 1,000 man hours worked, an extremely satisfactory state of affairs. By 1960 over 400 workers had been employed by Epihab and they had earned over one million dollars. In addition, 25 per cent had been placed in other companies. This venture represents a massive achievement which not only demonstrates that patients with epilepsy can be employed, but that they can use tools which most doctors would regard as foolhardy.

In the United Kingdom no such scheme exists but there are workshops of Remploy, run by the Department of Employment. Epileptic patients are included in the categories of disabled who are accepted by Remploy. Others may have diseases like disseminated sclerosis or be crippled as a result of an attack of poliomyelitis in their youth. Remploy has 7,800 employees of whom about 10 per cent have epilepsy. The epileptic workers have been found to be satisfactory and they are able to learn skills as quickly and efficiently as other groups. Similarly their accident and attendance records are not very different. In Sweden and Holland provision is made in sheltered workshops for those with epilepsy who cannot find suitable jobs in open industry, but to date only one organisation like Epihab exists in Europe. Started a few years ago under the guidance of Dr Risch, it is located at the village of Bethel near Hanover in Germany. It has so far made satisfactory progress in the rehabilitation of many patients, but the idea does not yet appear to be spreading.

It should be remembered that most patients with epilepsy will be employed in ordinary industry and only a small proportion needs special rehabilitation on the lines of Epihab or permanent sheltered workshop accommodation. Juul-Jensen of Denmark found that 5 per cent of his 969 patients required specialised employment help, while 75 per cent of the epileptic patients were able to find themselves work and continue to be employed satisfactorily.

The care of the epileptic person

The employer's point of view

In order to encourage employers to overcome their fears about employing epileptics in England, a pamphlet has been produced by the Department of Employment with the title *Employing Someone with Epilepsy*. It summarises the problems which may be encountered in taking on someone with fits, emphasising that some types of epilepsy do pose difficult problems for employment but many do not. However, the types of fits are highly individual, and even with severe epilepsy employment under normal industrial conditions is still possible. The pamphlet suggests that fear on the part of employers stems largely from outdated ideas on the nature of the condition and ignorance of recent medical advances. The wide variety of work an epileptic patient can do is emphasised. Some examples are the use of many hand tools and machine tools including certain lathes and presses. Epileptic people have been successfully employed in spray-painting bays, in stores and warehouses, and in offices as telephonists and receptionists, shorthand typists and clerks.

However, certain types of work are unsuitable, for example work with power-driven machinery, electrical switch gear and heating apparatus. Of course work with moving vehicles, as has already been said, is already excluded as well as traditionally forbidden "heights and ladders". Also epileptic people who may have a fit at work should not carry valuable, fragile objects. The Department pamphlet makes quite clear that this is not so much a list of don'ts as of ideas for guidance. Individual patients can often be found jobs with the help of Disabled Resettlement Officers who have special and local knowledge about factory work.

The settlement of an epileptic patient in a job requires not only the understanding and co-operation of the employer but also of other workers. To quote the pamphlet: "This is particularly important during the first few days of employment when the excitement and perhaps anxiety involved in taking up a new job may possibly bring on fits, which in most cases will diminish considerably in amount and severity when the worker has settled down and his confidence is regained. It is therefore important that a person with epilepsy has workmates who are not alarmed by an attack and know what to do if a fit should occur."

Quite often fits do not require a doctor to be called and many epileptic workers can resume their jobs very quickly after a fit. If of course fits become particularly frequent the patient has to be referred to his doctor.

If by chance an epileptic worker does injure himself at work this can be dealt with like any other industrial accident, and is covered by the National Insurance Act of 1946. Employers therefore do not have to worry about this.

Driving a car

Nowadays, the right to drive a car almost amounts to one of the freedoms of man. A patient with epilepsy, however, is not allowed to drive, and is thereby limited not only in work prospects, but in leisure activities. This ban used to apply equally to those who had not had an attack for ten years, as to those who were currently having many seizures. Now the position in Britain for the epileptic patient has changed somewhat, as we shall see.

No one will deny or expect that the man having many attacks a day should be allowed to drive. However, many patients with other types of illness drive and are equally liable to lose control of the car, for example those on heavy doses of tranquillising drugs, the diabetic patient on insulin, and those who have had a heart attack. All, like the epileptic person, can "black out". In addition the patient having infrequent epileptic attacks is certainly more in control than someone daily taking large quantities of alcohol; yet the person with fits is being penalised.

The result of this is that some patients may not disclose that they have seizures when they apply for a driving licence. This is, perhaps, a much more dangerous state of affairs than the issue of licences under strict control. Denial of a licence means that the patient with fits, who is often already insecure anyway, is even more undermined. This matter of driving licences was discussed at the 8th International Congress of Neurology in 1965, when a symposium was held on the subject. The views of neurologists from all over the world were heard, and there was a consensus of opinion that changes in the law were necessary in most countries. In particular they considered that patients with fits well controlled, on anti-convulsant medication, should have a licence granted to them.

However, to devise a foolproof system of controlled issue of licences is a problem; as we have seen the diagnosis of epilepsy itself is sometimes difficult. It is essential for this, as for other reasons, that the patient should be thoroughly investigated. Assuming that the diagnosis has been confirmed, information about the patient's seizure comes mainly from the patient himself, so that the physician has the greatest knowledge of his current seizure state. It would perhaps be an unfair burden to lay on the patient's own physician the decision whether to grant a licence or not. This could clearly undermine the relationship between a doctor and his patient. The situation could arise in which the patient might not report his fits, and might not seek medical help if he thought his licence would be revoked. Such masking of the facts would be undesirable and must be discouraged. An independent authority is obviously essential. In spite of these difficulties, in the state of Wisconsin in the United States a satisfactory procedure for the control of epileptic drivers' licences exists. This was planned by Dr Edward Schwabe. The physician looking after the patient certifies that he is free from attacks, a seizure-free period of two years usually being sufficient. A licence may then be granted for a six-month period, when after review it may be renewed for another six months and so on. If, however, the licence is refused, the patient's case can be studied by a board, on which there are two independent physicians qualified in the treatment of epilepsy. This arrangement has been in operation for ten years, during which time very few licences have been withdrawn, and few accidents have occurred as a result of fits.

Legislation came into effect in 1970 by which some people with epilepsy are allowed to drive in Britain. The main condition is that the person shall have had no attacks in the daytime for three years. The person applying for a licence has to answer questions about his epilepsy and give the Medical Officer of Health the name of his family doctor and other doctors who have treated him in the last three years. Reports are obtained from them, and the Medical Officer of Health advises the licensing authorities whether or not a licence to drive a car should be granted. It is subject to annual review. The Medical Committee of the British Epilepsy Association have prepared a pamphlet for family doctors and others on the subject. Clearly this is an important advance. It came about by pressure of both medical and lay opinion, but so far there is little information as to its effect.

Insurance of people with epilepsy

When the Driving Licence regulations were altered in Britain in 1970, epileptic drivers did have difficulty in obtaining insurance. Some companies are now more helpful. Insurance for accidents occurring at work presents few problems in Britain, but in the United States this is not true, though the situation is improving partly due to the efforts of Dr Frank Risch.

However, life insurance does present difficulty in Britain. It was impossible in the past to obtain even substandard life cover for epileptic sufferers. Now this can be achieved with less trouble, usually with a much higher premium than normal, especially for the first few years of the policy. The actuarial figures on which insurance companies base their calculations are ludicrously small, and the diagnostic categories vague. In addition, no allowances are made for modern methods of treatment. This whole area requires revision, so that the epileptic may get a fair deal in insurance. The same applies in many other areas of life. For example, he is unable at present to emigrate to many areas of the world. Enlightenment is advancing in some areas of social life, but progress is slow in many others.

The care of the epileptic person

Social services for epileptics

So far this book has explained what methods are available for helping epileptic patients within the framework of existing medical services. It is important now to consider what the ideal solution for the treatment of patients should be. Services are adequate neither for investigation nor for treatment, nor are the social services well enough developed to cope with the many patients who suffer from this chronic neurological disorder. Perhaps even more important, is that much is still unknown about epilepsy and research offers the only solution to the problem of fits. In the light of this it is interesting to consider the recommendation of the Cohen Committee on the care of epileptic patients. The Cohen Committee put forward twenty-three recommendations in 1956. If carried out, these would have revolutionised the care of the epileptic patient. However, in the fifteen years since these recommendations were made practically nothing has been done. The main recommendation was that Regional Hospital Boards should set up diagnostic and treatment units. These would have wards where epileptic patients could be diagnosed and stabilised on medication before returning home. The service would be run by a neurologist and a team of other doctors and ancillary staff, including radiologists, paediatricians and social workers.

Lord Hastings, speaking in the House of Lords in 1965 on services for the epileptic patient, said with great wisdom "without these diagnostic clinics and treatment centres it is virtually impossible to give the sufferer from epilepsy the proper chance that he should have to become assimilated into the community as a whole". The last part of the sentence is important; emphasis was placed, not on the hospital or epileptic colony for the patient, but on his assimilation into the community. This is a view which has already revolutionised the care of psychiatric patients.

The 1956 recommendations were not implemented, though, of course, there has been some improvement in the education of the public; even this has been very insufficient. Other recommendations of the Cohen Committee were that no child with epilepsy should be separated from his fellows by attending a special school unless it was essential. This could be avoided if the investigatory clinic for children with epilepsy and behaviour problems were suitably located.

It was suggested that epileptic colonies or centres, run by various private bodies, should with legislation be brought under the National Health Service, so that the chronic epileptic patient who requires more or less permanent supervision could be catered for. The care provided by the colonies could then be coupled with rehabilitation. The colony would no longer be a refuge, but a place from which assimilation into the community was possible. In a House of Lords debate, Baroness Summerskill deplored the fact that in a survey by Pond, about one-half of 282 patients suffering from epilepsy had not been referred to hospital for out-patient investigation and treatment, and said: "I welcome this debate very much because it will focus attention on the need for giving these patients expert treatment immediately the condition is revealed." The late Lord Brain also supported the view that diagnostic centres should be set up.

What then are the services provided in the United Kingdom and why are they unsatisfactory? The first person who sees the patient with epilepsy is the general practitioner. After taking a history of the condition from the patient and his relatives, he may examine him and prescribe anti-convulsant medication, and this he may do without referring him to a neurological specialist. Usually, however, most general practitioners rightly refer the patient to a consultant, or even for admission to a hospital where neurological investigations can be carried out. Investigations there usually include an EEG and X-rays. The results of these tests are sent back to the general practitioner with suggestions for treatment and further out-patient surveillance. In most instances there is nothing radically wrong with the care that epileptic patients receive, but they would certainly benefit from special clinics run by experts in the field, and in addition, such clinics could be the centre of research—

the activity on which the whole future planning of treatment and progress can be based.

So far most of what has been said applies to adult patients. When the patient is a child the hospital consultation is not usually carried out by a specialist in epilepsy, but by the paediatrician. At the age of eleven or so, the child is then transferred to another doctor, the adult neurologist. If neuro-surgery is contemplated, the patient is seen again by yet another doctor. Instead, the services could be organised in specialist units which would avoid this transfer of patients from one doctor to another. There are special clinics for diabetics and for alcoholics, so why should there not be special clinics for epileptic sufferers?

Some patients with epilepsy are cared for in special schools run by education authorities. Chronic patients are cared for in colonies or centres often run by voluntary agencies. Mentally subnormal epileptics are cared for by special services for the mentally retarded. Another group of chronic epileptic patients reside in mental hospitals and so the fragmentation of services continues. In none of these situations is the patient cared for by a specialist in epilepsy. At least none who has a full range of experience of epilepsy in different age groups and different situations could be graced with the term "epileptologists". The epileptic person has a series of medical, social, and sometimes psychological problems that need careful handling and all three fields could be cared for under the one roof. Services united in this way are not available in Britain.

In his book on *Living with Epileptic Seizures* Livingstone states: "my experience over the past twenty-six years has made it clear to me that many patients and also many physicians are unaware of the many services available for the epileptic patient":

1. Personal physicians and physicians who specialise in convulsive disorders.
2. Special epilepsy clinics.
3. Vocational and rehabilitation centres.
4. Lay (non-medical) organisations dealing with epilepsy.

5. Special hospital schools and institutions.

Things in Britain have by 1972 moved forward marginally. Because of pressure the Government set up yet another Committee to review the services for epileptic patients. The report of this Committee, "People with Epilepsy", was published in 1969, and has many excellent recommendations. Progress towards the implementation of these is reported in chapter XVII.

A specialist centre

The diagnosis and treatment of epilepsy are important steps for individual patients, and are best done at a specialist centre. However, this is not the only work of such a place, and there are other equally important aims. Dr William Lennox, at the Children's Medical Centre in Boston, said that training of doctors, carrying out of research, and the education of ancillary staff are all equally important. Only by training doctors in an environment where they see many and varied types of seizures and disorders, can they gain the experience they will require to run their own practices after leaving the centre. The doctor in training there will learn not only about the medical aspects of the condition but also about electro-encephalography and psychological testing. He will also learn about the social care of patients from those experienced in the field. A doctor so trained would not only be well informed, but will become interested in the care of epileptic patients.

Research is not just an academic discipline, it provides the fundamental knowledge on which everyday treatment of the patient can be based. For example the effects of a drug on all the organs of the body should be known before the dose can be adequately assessed. The staff at the Children's Medical Centre in Boston have been able to help, not only in research, but also in counselling parents and patients, for example on such matters as the advisability of having further children. Education is important too, not only for doctors, but also for patients, their parents, and the general public. When the public are aware of the difficulties from which the epileptic patient suffers, then such a patient is able to get a fair deal.

All these services require money, and this has to come partly from taxes and partly from private organisations. Investment of this money is required to improve the lot of those who suffer from epilepsy, and for straightforward economic benefits to the community. These patients who are often unable to find suitable employment, can with skilful handling be set to earning a living, as Dr Frank Risch has shown. Such techniques, according to Dr William Lennox, have already saved an estimated £14 million or 42 million dollars in the U.S.A.

International League against Epilepsy

To co-ordinate and promote the spread of knowledge about epilepsy the "International League Against Epilepsy" was founded in 1909. There were breaks during the 1914–18 and the 1939–45 wars, but afterwards the League was reformed and maintained periodic scientific meetings. This organisation has formed branches all over the world, including Europe and North and South America. Many distinguished doctors including some in Britain interested in epilepsy have served under its auspices and recently an international classification of epilepsy has been established. (See chapter XVII.) This, it is hoped, will enable doctors all over the world to pool their knowledge about epilepsy.

In addition to this there are other national and international non-medical groups.

The British Epilepsy Association

Much has been done in the last twenty years for those who have fits, but a great deal remains to be done. There is still throughout Great Britain an understandable reluctance to mention the word epilepsy, or for people to admit to having fits. It is this secrecy which hampers much of the work with epileptic patients. In addition it hinders the expansion of the British

Epilepsy Association. This latter has been in existence for twenty-one years and yet has an almost negligible membership of approximately 2,000 out of an estimated 250,000 in Great Britain, who have fits. There are understandably many people who do not wish to belong to an organisation but if 50 per cent of the sufferers from epilepsy were members, the association would be more powerful in helping to advance knowledge of epilepsy.

The association is a voluntary body and was founded in 1950 because particularly at that time many gaps existed in the state and local authority services. Clubs were founded so that people with epilepsy could meet their fellows and enjoy some sort of social life together. A welfare service dealt with many thousands of problems that could not be solved elsewhere and holidays were arranged for children with epilepsy. With the great expansion of local authority services, help and advice has become much more readily available and duplication of services is clearly wasteful and inefficient, so the emphasis has now changed and the Association co-operates with the state and local authorities wherever possible. It is working steadily to help to improve public understanding of epilepsy and to encourage research into the causes. However, it still maintains a full advice service with letters and telephone calls constantly coming in from members and non-members alike. Links are forged with Social Service Departments and workers all over the country who are in a position to give help and support to patients and relatives. In this way the efforts of voluntary and statutory bodies are co-ordinated.

Most local authorities now make holiday arrangements for the handicapped including those with epilepsy and, to help them in this undertaking, the British Epilepsy Association, with its specialised knowledge, is building up a list of suitable accommodation—i.e. hotels, guest houses and private houses where people with epilepsy and their families will be welcome. At the same time, it runs holidays annually for members of its clubs and a special holiday for severely handicapped epileptic children.

The educational aspects of the work are still somewhat hampered by lack of funds and staff, but it has become possible to extend the service throughout the whole country. Today, speakers are provided for meetings of all types—some formal, some informal, where the public can learn something of the history of epilepsy, its causes and the problems it can bring. Lectures are provided for many colleges of education so that teachers of the future will happily accept children with epilepsy in the classroom. Courses are organised for social workers, probation officers, health visitors, youth employment officers, disablement resettlement officers and others whose work may bring them into contact with epilepsy. These courses deal with medical and social aspects of epilepsy and the lecturers are all specialists in their own field. As a result of these lectures and the discussions which follow it is hoped to clear away misconceptions and present a clearer picture of the condition which embarrasses a quarter of a million people in this country.

There is a great need for education among both employers and employed. There are many professions from which people with epilepsy are virtually excluded because they cannot be accepted into the pension fund. Banks are notoriously difficult in this connection. Some firms are beginning to show a more helpful approach by reviewing their schemes so that applicants may be considered as individuals and not categorically rejected because of the label "epilepsy". These firms realise that the mere rigidity of superannuation and pension schemes debars people with excellent qualifications from jobs in which they would do well. The education of other employers and their personnel is the only hope. Patient, painstaking endeavour will slowly overcome prejudice—there seems to be no convenient short cut to enlightenment. It is heartening to remember how short a time ago tuberculosis was regarded with the same horror. People cannot act better until they know better!

Get ordinary people to understand about epilepsy, and one hopes the difficulties of employment will lessen. Conquer that and at once there emerges the problem of accommodation. Sometimes school and training have been gone through successfully; a sympathetic employer has the right and sensible attitude; the job is waiting; but accommodation is missing. No one wants to share a flat, no one wants to let a flat, no landlady wants a paying guest with fits. The answer might be the establishment of hostels for epileptics, but this would at once single them out as people who have to be isolated, segregated—a class apart. The man or woman with epilepsy is a person in his own right whose brain now and then, for some obscure reason, has outbursts of electrical overactivity; otherwise he is no different from his fellow.

A more enlightened understanding of this underlying fact by the general public will serve to overcome these obstacles, which frequently create difficulties for epileptic people who are trying to find a job and somewhere to live. It is this challenge which is being faced by the British Epilepsy Association in its efforts to bring more knowledge to all those who have it in their power to help, whether in the role of employer, colleague, landlady, flat-mate or simply as a fellow citizen.

Ignorance about epilepsy is not confined to this country. Social workers and doctors in most countries are agreed that it is more difficult to mend the public attitude to epilepsy than to provide medical care. Hence the International Bureau for Epilepsy was founded; the British Epilepsy Association is a member of this Bureau which now has branches throughout the world to fight for the social rights of epileptic sufferers, for example the right to have insurance and driving licences, etc. Immigration is another example, for many countries specifically bar people with epilepsy. Consider the three following statements:

Australia. "The Migration Act passed by the Australian Parliament in 1958 provides that persons suffering from certain diseases including epilepsy shall in general be prohibited from migrating to Australia. There is provision for special entry permits to be granted, but in practice such permits are issued only in unusual circumstances on the authority of the Immigration Authorities in Canberra. Epilepsy is one of the diseases in question. It may therefore be taken that persons known to be suffering from epilepsy will not usually be eligible to enter Australia."

Brazil: "According to Brazilian legislation epileptics are not accepted as immigrants to Brazil."

Uruguay: "One of the requisites for a permanent visa into Uruguay is a medical certificate, issued by the Consulate Doctor to the effect that the applicant does not suffer from epilepsy among other illnesses."

The International Bureau is trying to spread enlightenment in this and many other fields. The British Epilepsy Association produces films and publishes articles in the Press carrying on the work of enlightenment. Leaflets and booklets are always available for those wanting to know more about epilepsy in general or to study some special aspect—while the magazine *The Candle*, published twice a year, carries topical articles by specialists from all over the world.

Education is important but research is vital, to answer the questions: What is epilepsy? What causes it? Why do some people get it and not others? Why in this day of supposedly uninhibited attitudes does the very word "epilepsy" bring a look of startled horror? Why will people accept most things but not epilepsy? Why is it feared? What causes this subconscious recoil? These are things which are not known, and which must be investigated. Unfortunately the amount available for research into one of man's oldest afflictions is infinitesimal by comparison with the millions spent in solving the mysteries of travel in space. An Epilepsy Research Fund was established in 1968. So far, almost thirty grants have been made to hospitals and individual doctors and sociologists. Subjects investigated range from the ill effects of anti-convulsants on children to the psychology of stigma.

The Association provides a comprehensive service of information dealing with all aspects of epilepsy but most particularly with the social aspects. It undertakes the work involved in a national programme of both generalised and specialised education and information. A panel of trained speakers is available for meetings throughout the country.

Those who would like to know more of the work of the British Epilepsy Association should write to:

The Director
British Epilepsy Association
3–6 Alfred Place
London, WC1E 7ED

Details can be obtained about membership of the Association, and its work, its clubs, and its branches in Sheffield, Merseyside, Birmingham and Portsmouth.

Information about epilepsy in other countries can be obtained from the:

Secretary General
International Bureau for Epilepsy
3–6 Alfred Place
London, WC1E 7ED

CHAPTER FIFTEEN

Marriage and Pregnancy

Marriage

MARRIAGE is one of the central goals of life for many people. However, the epileptic child may sometimes be over-protected by his parents, for example, not be allowed to play with neighbours' children or to invite them home. As a result isolation begins early in life. This may continue as an adolescent and adult, so that the step of courtship and marriage may be much more difficult for the person with fits. There is, of course, no reason for the doctor to dissuade the patient from marriage. The stability of marriage is usually good and may lead to a decrease in the frequency of attacks. However, it is most important that the non-epileptic partner is told about epilepsy before marriage, because if this is not thoroughly discussed at that time, it may cause difficulties afterwards.

There are no medical grounds for forbidding marriage; but in Sweden, until recently, and still to the present time (information complete to 1965) in four states of the U.S.A., laws prevent an epileptic from marrying. West Virginia forbids epileptics to marry under any circumstances, while North Carolina requires that sterilization (see below) is carried out before a marriage licence can be issued. In fact, in some states it is a criminal offence for epileptics to marry. This "criminal activity" includes not only the "happy couple", but also the official who carries out the ceremony! Another aspect of the laws to control epileptic sufferers is shown by an extract from the *Daily Telegraph* of the 11th October, 1965, which mentions a woman from England, who was forbidden to join her fiancée in Hartford, Connecticut. "It took a special act of Congress to permit this," the correspondent continues; "American law bans the entry of an epileptic for permanent residence." After the passing of the special act of Congress, the couple were able to be married and the law was amended soon after.

In the past, epilepsy was regarded as a strongly inherited disease and so eugenic laws were passed in order to prevent the birth of "tainted offspring". Now that more information is available suggesting that inheritance plays a relatively small part in the causation of fits, the laws are clearly not only outdated, but also barbaric. Another outdated law still exists in fourteen states of the U.S.A. which calls for the sterilisation of epileptic people. Fortunately, though this law still exists, it has probably not been enforced for many years. In the fourteen states affected by these laws the sterilisation is under the control of the administration of the state institutions who may quite legally sterilise epileptic inmates. In two states, North Carolina and Utah, non-institutionalised epileptic patients may also be sterilised. Iowa also allows sterilisation of people who would be likely to inherit an epileptic tendency. It will be seen from the following section that the interpretation of this statute would be extremely difficult.

The inheritance of epilepsy

In the past it was considered that all types of epilepsy were inherited and there was great fear in the minds of patients that their children might develop fits. Fortunately these fears were exaggerated and, though epilepsy may be inherited, the risk is much less than previously considered. It must, however, be made clear at the outset that much still remains to be learnt about the inheritance of epilepsy. Some types may have a relatively strong tendency to be inherited and in others (this is true of many instances of symptomatic epilepsy) inheritance is unlikely to play any significant part at all.

Recently doctors, notably at the Hospital for Sick Children at Great Ormond Street in London, have started a "genetics clinic". Here people may go for advice about the possible inheritance of some rare diseases. This type of clinic obviously needs to be extended more widely, so not only can parents be given advice, but also more can be learnt about the mechanisms and intricacies of inheritance. Certainly if someone is contemplating getting married to an epileptic patient they should seek to ascertain the possibility of a child of theirs suffering from epilepsy. Some problems in this field will now be explained, as they apply to a hypothetical couple, one of whom suffers from fits and one who does not.

This couple who intend to marry ask the doctor "What is the likelihood of our children having epilepsy?" An answer to this question can only be given accurately when the type of epilepsy from which the individual suffers has been determined. On some occasions it is discovered during the investigation of the attacks that they are not epileptic in nature at all, but relate to disease of the heart or blood vessels. If however, the diagnosis of epilepsy is established and, for example, a brain scar is discovered (perhaps as a result of a road accident) then the children of such an individual are most unlikely to inherit epilepsy.

However, the question of inheritance is usually raised by someone who suffers from epilepsy in which no scar nor disease of the brain can be detected by investigation. This is the type in which inheritance does play a part, and a considerable number of studies have been carried out to investigate the likelihood of fits in the children of such epileptic parents. Dr Kurt Alström from Sweden examined a group of 897 adult patients, and found that the incidence of epilepsy among their relatives was only 1·5 per cent. Dr William Lennox in the U.S.A. studied a larger group of 200,000 relatives of adult patients. He found that 3·2 per cent of the relatives had epilepsy. However, if those who suffered only occasional attacks in childhood during feverish illnesses were excluded, the figure was reduced to 1·6 per cent almost identical to that of Dr Alström.

As in other inherited diseases, information has been gained by examination of twins. The method is ingenious. The twins are divided into two groups, one containing the identical twins, and the other, the non-identical twins. In the group of identical twins, genetic inheritance of each twin of a pair is the same, because the two individuals result from a single fertilised egg. Non-identical twins, like other non-twin members of the family, are of similar but not identical inheritance. Information is then gathered on the upbringing of the twins. This includes whether or not the twins have been reared together in the same family, or in separate homes. In this way it is possible to compare the importance of both nature (or inheritance) and/or nurture (environment) and assess the roles of each. Dr William Lennox managed to collect 225 pairs of twins, about half of which were identical. Sixty per cent of the identical twin pairs both had epilepsy, while in the group of non-identical twins the figure was about 15 per cent. Lennox concluded that inheritance is important in the causation of epilepsy.

However, there are some other matters to take into account when giving advice about the likelihood of children developing epilepsy. Sometimes epilepsy arises in families in which no members have ever had it before. The chances of this are small, about 0·5 per cent, that is about 1 in every 200 children born. Another point is that certain other common diseases are also inherited. Diabetes is an example. The children of affected diabetic parents are twice as likely to develop diabetes as the children of epileptic parents to develop epilepsy.

Our hypothetical couple, one of whom has epilepsy, is told that the risk of a child of theirs developing fits is about three or four times greater than for non-epileptic parents, i.e. about a 1·5 per cent chance compared with 0·5 per cent.

One point must be remembered. The effect of epilepsy in a woman is different from that in a man. Fits may affect motherhood in women (see below), and possibly "bread-winning" in the man. It is better that these problems are discussed before marriage rather than left to create difficulties after.

When, however, both parents have epilepsy or it runs in the family of one of them, the risk of offspring developing the condition is at least twice that for the hypothetical couple. The advice must then be guarded, and requires the services of an expert in the field who makes use of E E G examinations of both parents.

Pregnancy

Pregnancy will result as readily from the union of an epileptic as a non-epileptic couple, as fertility has not been shown to be affected by epilepsy. The pregnant mother with fits must continue to take anti-convulsant medication throughout pregnancy. Fortunately this appears to have no adverse effects on the unborn child. Sometimes fits during pregnancy occur as frequently as before pregnancy. Sometimes they are more frequent and just occasionally, some women are fortunate in losing their attacks altogether, though they usually recur after the birth of the child.

At the end of pregnancy, labour will begin and proceed normally as for the non-epileptic mother, and the birth is quite likely to be uneventful. However, the mother is best advised not to breast-feed the baby, unless her fits are well controlled, because a fit occurring during feeding, might result in injury to the baby. Another reason for advising against breast-feeding concerns anti-convulsant drugs. These leave the blood stream and reach the mother's breast milk, so they may cause a "drugged baby". Otherwise, the child can be brought up like any other.

In summary it appears that there is little justification for laws to prevent marriage, or to enforce sterilisation on epileptic sufferers. In some types of epilepsy there is a risk of inheritance and though many studies with identical and non-identical twins, for example, have been carried out, much remains to be investigated. For the sufferer who contemplates marriage, professional advice should be sought. In this way the exact risk involved in a particular marriage can be found.

CHAPTER SIXTEEN

The prevention of fits

Prevention is of prime importance in modern medicine. For example, the infectious disease diphtheria has been controlled by immunisation and is almost extinct in Britain. Prevention is also important in non-infectious diseases, for example, early diagnosis may reduce mortality in patients with cancer. Is it possible, then, to apply preventive measures to epilepsy? From the evidence concerning inheritance (see chapter XV) there seems little point in controlling marriage of epileptic patients or carrying out sterilisation, since the risks are small. However, there are ways in which epilepsy can be prevented, as recently put forward by Taylor and Bower. One that they emphasise is the prevention of damage to the brain by injury or infection.

Importance of head injuries

If the frequency of head injuries could be reduced, many cases of epilepsy could be prevented. It is estimated that in the course of a year in Britain some 250,000 people suffer from a head injury, and about 100,000 are admitted to hospital. Of these perhaps 5 per cent die as a result of their injury, and a similar number probably develop epilepsy, though there is disagreement among doctors as to the exact figure. This certainly

143

applies to those who, as the result of an injury at work or on the road, are "knocked out" and possibly sustain a fracture of the skull (see figure 16). If however, the condition is more serious the scalp is lacerated, the bone broken and the brain damaged, as might occur in some of the severe forms of car accidents or in injuries with bullets or shrapnel during wartime,

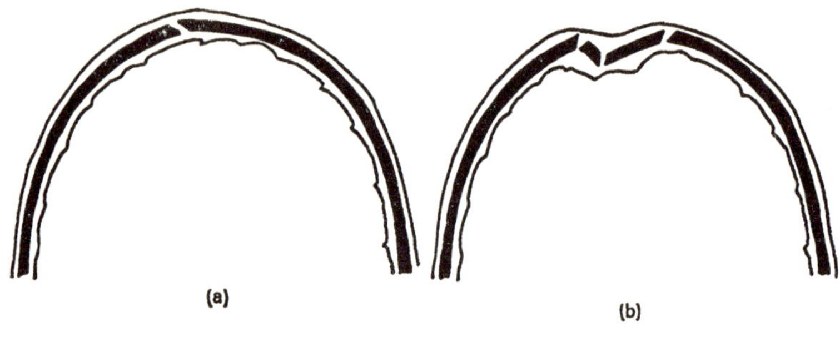

FIG. 16.

(a) A fracture of the skull without displacement of the fragments.
(b) A fracture of the skull with depression of the fragments. These may damage the brain and cause epileptic fits subsequently.

then the incidence of epilepsy in such patients is much higher than 5 per cent. In fact as many as 40–50 per cent of these may develop epilepsy. Sometimes fits begin fairly soon after the accident, at other times not for many years. The E E G may help to decide whether the person is likely to develop fits, but this is not always the case.

Sometimes the patient who has epilepsy after head injury suffers from major attacks, but on other occasions the patient experiences focal fits. These often are preceded by a warning, and quite commonly the temporal lobe, which lies on the under surface of the brain, is vulnerable to damage during the head injury and is the site of origin of the abnormal electrical discharge. Fortunately, epilepsy following head injury can often be controlled by drugs and on a few occasions it is possible to remove the scarred area of brain at a surgical operation.

The prevention of epilepsy in this context means limiting not only accidents on the road, but also those in the factory or on the building site. There should be even more strenuous efforts to encourage motor cyclists to wear crash helmets and motorists to use safety belts. In addition factory conditions must be improved, so that accidents are reduced there. On building sites, particularly when high buildings are being erected, workers on the ground should wear helmets, and the same is true in the shipyard. It was there that an interesting survey of the EEG changes immediately following head injury was carried out. As soon as a workman was hit by a falling object, his EEG was taken and valuable information was obtained about the immediate electrical disturbance that takes place.

Improved care of mothers during pregnancy and during delivery of the child have already produced a marked decrease in epilepsy. Care of infants and young children who are particularly vulnerable to infections of the brain like meningitis can also help to reduce brain damage and epilepsy. These conditions require prompt treatment to prevent the formation of scars on the surface and in the brain. These scars cause irritation of the surrounding nerve cells and a focus from which epileptic discharges may arise. One other condition which in itself does not seem particularly serious may lead to temporal lobe epilepsy in adult life: the febrile convulsion (see p. 79). Some doctors now treat these convulsions very rigorously, giving a prolonged course of anti-convulsants even after a single fit. More research is obviously required on this topic.

Fits arise spontaneously in families whose parents are free of the inheritance of epilepsy. This may be due to spontaneous changes in the genes which are responsible for the inheritance of satisfactory as well as unsatisfactory characteristics. Undesirable changes in genes, or mutations as they are called, may be brought about also by exposure to X-rays and atomic radiation. There is the possibility, though at present a theoretical one, that epilepsy would increase, like some other disorders, over the next few generations as a result of the action of radioactive fall-out.

It is therefore important that this possible source of damage to the genes is reduced or eliminated.

Unfortunately, the prevention of epilepsy is still in its infancy and apart from the control of head injuries, relatively little can be done at present.

Do fits get better?

There is a tendency as the person gets older for all types of fits to die away. Sometimes they cease entirely and, in other instances, they become infrequent, perhaps as few as one or two per year. *Petit mal* attacks usually begin in early childhood, and by the age of twenty years will have ceased altogether, or have been replaced by *grand mal* fits. These latter convulsive attacks, though longer in duration, are usually less frequent and are often responsive to anti-convulsant medication. In their turn, *grand mal* attacks become less frequent and may disappear completely. Temporal lobe fits, usually more common in adults than children, nevertheless with increasing age also become less frequent and may stop altogether.

A detailed recent study on the outlook for epileptic patients has been made by Rodin, but the experience of Livingstone is like that of others in the field and gives a broad general view. He suggests that complete control of seizures can be obtained in about 60 per cent of patients, and in another 25 per cent the frequency of seizures is greatly reduced. There remains, however, a small group in whom the frequency of attacks is, unfortunately, not greatly influenced by medication, but as newer substances become available they too can be helped.

Over the past twenty-five years there has been a great change in the treatment of epilepsy. At that time bromide and phenobarbitone only were available, but new medications have been introduced for all types of attacks. The search continues for newer and more efficient drugs, so there is no need for patients or relatives to despair, when fits are not well controlled, for other medications appear every so often.

Injuries during fits

One of the worries the patient and his family may have, even though not overtly expressed, is the fear that death will occur during an attack. Such an occurrence during a single fit, even though it may be a convulsion, is extremely rare. Status epilepticus, on the other hand, carries a considerable mortality. Perhaps almost as worrying is the fear that a serious injury may occur during an attack. When patients have an aura, they may be able to use this brief warning to avoid danger. Then again some patients without auras may have other early signs of an impending attack, for example, the turning of the head, at which the parents or relatives may take similar precautions. It is true that injuries *can* happen during attacks, but serious injuries are relatively rare. Of course, children who are always damaging their heads or chins in uncontrolled attacks should be protected, for example, by a helmet. One other important fact mentioned earlier that has to be explained is that fits are less frequent in periods of alertness. They rarely occur at work, but often occur in states of drowsiness. Statistics of accidents at work show that epileptic sufferers have almost the same accident rate as their more fortunate colleagues. It might be thought that crossing the road would be dangerous for people suffering from fits, but an epileptic convulsion in the middle of the road is an extremely rare event. The most generally dangerous place is the home. An epileptic person may have an attack and fall against an electric fire, for example. During the unconscious state following the attack, he cannot feel the pain of the burn and does not pull himself away. Such burns are likely to be very severe, often requiring treatment by a plastic surgeon.

Mortality in those with epilepsy

It may be asked, "Does the epileptic person live as long as someone without epilepsy" or "Does he finally die of complications of epilepsy or in a fit?" Information on both of these topics is scanty, but surveys carried out by Schwabe and Otto in the State of Wisconsin, U.S.A., in 1953, showed that 0·2 per cent of all deaths were related to epilepsy, a figure that compared with about 2 per cent for diabetes. In fact, 79 epileptic persons were found to have died in the Wisconsin survey; 60 per cent died of causes unrelated to epilepsy, and the remainder were as a consequence of an accident in a fit, or status epilepticus. Alström found in Sweden that the mortality in a large group of epileptic patients hardly exceeded that of the general population.

The mortality of patients with epilepsy has also fallen considerably over the past fifty years. In the United States in 1905 the figure was about 18 per 200,000 of the population, but by 1955 the figure had fallen to just below 3 per 200,000 of the population. This compared with a drop in death rate for all causes from about 16 per 200,000 to 9 per 200,000. This clearly indicates the relatively improved position of epileptic patients, a trend which should continue with increasing knowledge and better medical care. The rare condition of status epilepticus is still the most important single cause of death for epileptic patients, though very occasionally death does occur after a single fit. There are also isolated reports of death by drowning and there does appear to be a risk of suicide in some epileptic patients. The information on these aspects, however, is still incomplete.

Brain damage caused by fits

A question often asked is, "Do fits damage the brain?" In spite of the frequent attacks the brain of an epileptic patient when examined by the pathologist in the post mortem room shows little evidence of damage as a result. In other conditions, for example following strokes, there may be wasting of an area of the brain or distortion of the normal pattern, but with epilepsy no such abnormalities are usually seen. However, during status epilepticus the cells are starved of oxygen and this may lead to severe damage of the brain. Such damage is manifested by areas of wasting and softening. It is to minimise this brain

148

damage that status epilepticus must be treated quickly and completely.

There is another type of evidence that can be examined to show whether fits are damaging to the brain or not. In the course of the studies of identical twins with one epileptic and the other normal (see chapter IX), their intelligence quotients were tested by psychologists. It was found that the intelligence of the twins were similar, indicating that the brain was not damaged by fits. Nevertheless it must be admitted that some patients who have very frequent fits (usually convulsions) do deteriorate mentally for no apparent cause; such a condition, it should be emphasised, is uncommon.

To sum up: the only way we can hope to prevent epilepsy at present is to protect the head from injuries from the moment of birth onwards. Fits of whatever kind are controlled completely in about two-thirds of patients by the use of anti-convulsants. Even when fits are frequent, death is rare except in cases of status epilepticus.

CHAPTER SEVENTEEN

Growing points

OUR UNDERSTANDING of epilepsy is still fragmentary. So much so that some doctors would say we know very little at all about it. What then are the problems to be solved and how are they to be studied?

One of the most important is how fits are caused. We know a few things about this but not enough yet to give us the solution. Some of the questions which remain unanswered in this connection are as follows. Of the people who have head injuries as a result of motor accidents, why do only a small proportion develop fits? It might be because of the severity of the injury or the particular part of the skull or brain injured; it might be related to an epileptic inheritance in the family. We know the possible explanations but, so far, we have no way of being certain which applies to a particular accident.

Another problem is how damaged brain cells give rise to epileptic discharges? Something is known about the spread of epileptic discharges once they develop but their origin is still shrouded in mystery. There is a further difficulty. Everyone has the ability to have a fit if the provocative stimulus is great enough. It may require, in many, a considerable electric shock or the injection of a convulsant drug. Nevertheless, the problem remains—why do some people have fits with little provocation and others require a much larger stimulus to produce a fit? One possible explanation would be that people who do not suffer from epilepsy have a suppressor mechanism, while those with fits do not. So far this mechanism has eluded scientists, though it was hoped that gamma-amino-butyric acid was the "missing link". Nevertheless, research in progress is helping to clarify many aspects of the matter. For those who wish to study this in more detail, bibliographical details are available at the end of the book.

Classification of fits

The fundamental issues of causation were well appreciated by an international group under the chairmanship of Professor Henri Gastaut, set up by the International League against Epilepsy in 1964. Their terms of reference were to propose a comprehensive classification of epileptic seizures so that doctors all over the world might use it and allow more accurate exchange of information. It is clearly of little general value for one doctor to report the treatment of a certain type of fit with a new drug, if elsewhere this type of fit is not recognised. The international group observed, however, that all attempts at the classification of epileptic seizures were hampered by "limited knowledge of the underlying pathological process within the brain". They continued that "any classification must of necessity be a tentative one and will be subject to change with every advance in scientific understanding of epilepsy". It was one of the first times that a group of individuals rather than a single individual had attempted this task in relation to epilepsy, though of course international agreement has been reached in other medical and scientific fields. This classification represents a fundamental step in research which will allow a more valuable exchange of knowledge than has ever been possible before. This will eventually benefit the individual patient in countries as remote from each other as England and Japan, Uruguay and India.

In earlier chapters simpler and less adequate classifications and terminology have been used. These are still in general use, though as discussions and improvements of the international classification proceed it is hoped that this will replace the older systems completely.

Table II

International Classification of Epileptic Seizures

Summary Form of Classification

1. Partial seizures or seizures beginning locally:
   A. With elementary symptomatology (motor, sensory or autonomic symptoms);
   B. With complex symptomatology (automatism, ideational, psychosensory, psychomotor, etc., symptoms);
   C. Generalised seizures with local onset. (N.B. All partial seizures can develop into generalised seizures, sometimes so rapidly that the local features may not be observable.)
2. Generalised seizures or seizures without local onset:
   A. Absence of differing form and duration, including "absence status". Absences may occur alone, or in combination with myoclonic jerks, or with increase or loss of postural tone, or with automatisms.
   B. Generalised convulsive seizures, in the form of tonic, clonic, tonicoclonic and/or myoclonic attacks.
3. Unilateral or predominantly unilateral seizures (tonic and/or clonic) in children.
4. Erratic seizures in new-born.
5. Unclassified seizures. This includes all seizures which cannot be classified because of inadequate or incomplete data.

The summary form of classification in Table II divides fits into two. First, those that begin locally, and second, those that do not.

The first group, which begin in what is called an epileptic focus, are sometimes called "partial seizures". These would include those already described as Jacksonian fits, and temporal lobe fits, as well as adversive and psychomotor seizures; about this latter term there is particular disagreement which will be discussed later. In addition, this group of seizures includes some generalised convulsions or *grand mal* beginning with an aura.

The second group are without evidence of a "focal" beginning; they have no aura. Some forms of *grand mal* are in this group, also *petit mal* or *absence*. Unfortunately two other groups are needed for fits of childhood which are less easily classified, and finally there is a group of unclassified seizures, principally because the information given is inadequate to place them accurately in any of the other groups.

In spite of its apparent completeness, this classification of the different types of fits is the subject of great controversy, and at least one doctor in Britain has said that it would take a further ten years' study before a satisfactory working classification of epilepsy could be put forward. After that, it would probably take as long again to put it into action. As time passes and knowledge increases it will be possible to see if this brave attempt at international co-operation has been worth while.

Research

Research is essential to fill in the vast gaps in our knowledge of epilepsy. William Lennox linked the importance of research to the education of doctors, nurses, psychologists and others. He felt that, for good research to be carried out, accurate observation was required, and this needed careful training. Such training, however, requires not only hard work from the participants, but also foresight and ideas, perhaps most important of all. Research programmes have been limited by lack of money, so only limited success has been achieved so far. However, there are many areas in which fundamental research into epilepsy is being undertaken, with a measure of success.

Animal research. One possible method of investigation involves the use of animals. It may seem that production of epileptic fits in animals is not humane, but for many years animals have been used for the testing of anti-epileptic drugs before they were administered to human patients. There is no other way that they can be tested, as it is clearly unethical to give untried and potentially toxic medications to patients, because such substances may even cause death. Animals can also be used in other ways to clarify the effects of epilepsy on the brain itself and on mental processes and behaviour in general. Fits may be induced either by electrical or by chemical means, and these two groups of experiments will be described separately.

Rats are often used for experimental studies involving the induction of fits by electrical stimulation. An electrode is implanted in one area of the brain and a standard electrical current is applied to it daily for a standard period of, for example, one minute. Animals treated in this way will eventually have a convulsion, but this never occurs in the first few days of stimulation, however powerful the stimulating current. Hence it appears that the passage of an electrical current changes the cells in the brain in some way which allows convulsions to take place more easily.

It is found that some areas of the brain are sensitive to the electrical stimulation and others less so. For example, an area called the amygdala deep in the temporal lobe is particularly sensitive; whereas some areas show no convulsive response even after 200 days of regular stimulation. Detailed studies have been carried out on the cells near the tip of the stimulating electrode, and it has been found that they show patterns of activity quite unlike those seen in normal brain cells. How these cells "impose" abnormal firing on the rest of the brain so that a convulsion results, is still unknown. In addition, whether these experiments carried out on rats are applicable to man is also uncertain, but they suggest hypotheses that can be tested further.

Sometimes in these stimulation experiments changes occur in other cells remote from the stimulated region. Such a phenomenon does occur in man and is called a "mirror focus". If a marked discharge is found in one temporal lobe after a few years it may be noted that epileptic activity is arising from the opposite temporal lobe in the other hemisphere of the brain. This development of a mirror focus has profound effects on the patient, who not only has frequent fits but other marked changes, for example in memory. Animal experiments are being carried out to investigate this particularly unfortunate development. If it were known why such a mirror focus develops and how it can be prevented, many patients would lead happier lives. So far it has not been possible to predict in which patients such a focus will develop. If prediction were possible, then treatment by operation would be effective. Animal experiments are being carried out to elucidate this particular problem, and for this and other studies chemical rather than electrical induction of fits is employed.

In animals certain chemicals are applied to the outer surface of the brain (the cortex); after a latent period of a few weeks the damaged cells begin to produce an epileptic discharge, and the animals may develop epilepsy. A wide variety of chemicals has been tried and the most effective have been cobalt and aluminium hydroxide. Cobalt is particularly reliable in producing fits in rats. In monkeys it is much more difficult to apply the correct amount, and the animals either develop very severe epilepsy or do not develop fits at all. In addition, cobalt is known to be very toxic. It causes widespread damage to the brain cells as well as producing epilepsy. This would obviously make the effects of epilepsy *per se* difficult to determine. Aluminium hydroxide, on the other hand, has been found to be very effective in producing fits in monkeys. A small amount of aluminium hydroxide is either injected into the brain or placed on its surface. This almost invariably results in the development of focal epileptic fits. Sometimes, however, these fits can only be "picked up" by the EEG, as there is apparently no change in the monkey's behaviour.

Because of the reliability of this substance in producing fits, many research workers have been able to do controlled studies to determine the effects of abnormal electrical activity on memory and learning. In most studies the animals are taught two or more problems, for example to distinguish between a circle and a cone. They then have some of the aluminium hydroxide placed on a particular area of their brain. When the fit develops—this is usually measured by the EEG—they are then required to remember the problems that they had previously been taught. In addition they are also required to learn some new problems (still while they are having fits or are having abnormal electrical activity in the brain as shown by the EEG recording).

Their scores on these problems are compared with monkeys who have had no aluminium hydroxide applied. The majority of results show that those animals with epilepsy can remember as well as normal animals, but that their attempts at learning new problems while they are having fits is impaired.

These results are also, interestingly enough, quite different from those obtained if a comparable area of cortex is excised, for then the animals show a loss in both learning and memory.

Although aluminium hydroxide produces somewhat less damage than cobalt, further studies would be necessary to determine whether it is the fits *per se* in such monkeys which are causing losses in learning, or whether the aluminium hydroxide alone or in combination with the fits is producing enough damage to account for such losses (see Moffett et al.).

Local freezing of the surface of the brain is another technique that has been used for producing fits. This has been found to be reliable, but unfortunately the fits are much more shortlived than with either cobalt or aluminium hydroxide, which means that there is insufficient time to determine their effects on learning and memory.

Until now animals have been used in the routine testing of anti-convulsant drugs to make sure they are not toxic. A recent observation by Killam and Naquet of Marseilles suggested a new test method. They observed that baboons will have epileptic fits if exposed to the rapidly flashing light used at present in EEG laboratories. In addition, spike and wave discharges can be seen on the EEG trace at the same time as the fits. A variety of drugs were given to the baboons before they were exposed to the flash, and it was observed that some "blocked" the appearance of EEG discharge and the occurrence of fits. Two drugs were found to be effective in this way: phenobarbitone, used in the treatment of patients with epilepsy for many years, and diazepam (valium), which was introduced more recently. The final place of this technique in the study of drugs is not established, but preliminary results suggest it may be of great value in the search for new anti-convulsant medications.

Advances in electro-encephalography

Another field of research concerns the use of more advanced electro-encephalographic apparatus. Earlier, it was mentioned that Berger's EEG apparatus was very limited; he was able to record from only one part of the brain at a time. However, soon after his first reports, many doctors all over the world began carrying out similar studies. Grey Walter in England was among the first to take up this technique, realising that it had potential application not only for medical diagnosis but also for research of a fundamental nature into the workings of the brain. He was able to show with a roomful of apparatus that abnormal waves arose from a brain tumour when there were no other means by which the tumour could be detected. In addition, the exact location of the tumour in the brain could also be determined.

This early exciting era of electro-encephalography was followed by the 1939–45 war, when vast technical strides were made in electronics. Since that time apparatus has decreased in size, and it is technically possible now to reduce the whole EEG machine from the size of a suitcase to little more than a matchbox.

This small piece of equipment could be attached to the patient's head so that he was able to walk around and carry out any ordinary activity while his brain waves were being recorded. These could either be stored in a minute tape-recorder, also on the head, or transmitted by the equipment to some distant point (telemetry) where the waves could be written out as the usual ink trace on paper. Clearly in this way it would be possible to record an EEG for the whole day. If a patient had frequent epileptic attacks, the record of the EEG and observations of the patient could be accurately compared. However, this rapid technical advance has been little used so far by doctors, partly because of their unfamiliarity with the equipment, and partly because of the cost. However, the early results of the application of this technique to the study of epilepsy are beginning to emerge in 1972 (see Geier). They indicate that there is a complex relationship between the occurrence of EEG abnormality and overt fits. Sometimes what appears to be a fit to the observer is not associated with EEG abnormality, and vice versa. Clearly more studies of this kind will be necessary, but already there is enough evidence to suggest that this should prove a valuable method of studying patients having frequent attacks, in order to determine just which is the best drug in the treatment of their epilepsy.

The use of computers. Another recent technical advance important in the study of epilepsy from both the clinical and electro-encephalographic point of view is the computer. Essentially it allows vast amounts of information to be manipulated more easily. Consider the careful study, which will be described later, in which a sample of Isle of Wight schoolchildren aged 9–11, were examined by neurologists and psychologists. There were already details of their previous medical history and their school records. Then there were hundreds of items of information noted at the time of the medical and psychological examination. To deal with this information by hand would take years. However, by careful coding of the information, and by punching it on cards or paper tape, this could be fed into a computer and processed much more quickly. In fact, in a few minutes tables could be produced showing the number with epileptic fits, asthma and other disorders, or the ones backward in reading, arithmetic, or those who had previous severe illnesses or had been in hospital for long periods. The computer is thus valuable for rapid processing of medical and other data, and for finding relationships among apparently isolated items.

Computers are also valuable aids in analysis of the EEG. This has been less well developed but involves the recording of the EEG in the form of either paper tape or magnetic tape, of a kind similar to that used in ordinary tape recorders. The computer deals quickly with the information and indicates, for example, which area of the brain is involved in an epileptic process.

At the Brain Research Institute in Los Angeles a computer technique is being developed in conjunction with "depth electrode studies". These types of study (mentioned earlier in connection with temporal lobe surgery) consist essentially of inserting fine wire electrodes deep into the brain, through a small hole made in the skull of the patient by a neuro-surgeon. These electrodes may be left in place for days so that the spike activity characteristic of epilepsy can be recorded. If electrodes are located in various parts of the temporal lobe, the most actively discharging part, i.e. that part emitting the greatest amount of abnormal epileptic activity, can be determined. The next stage would then be to remove that area by operation or possibly by passing a strong electrical current down the electrode, a method which will often destroy a localised area of brain successfully. These techniques are in their infancy, and many years of research will be necessary before their final place in treatment is assured.

One other investigatory technique, using a small computer and requiring no neuro-surgery, has become available in the past few years. It is based on the principle that the brain produces electrical discharges in response to stimuli such as a sound in the ear or a flash of light in the eyes. The responses to these are usually small and difficult to pick out in the E E G. However, the "averaging computer" is able to carry this out automatically and show different types of response with different stimuli. This technique has been applied by Bablouzian and colleagues to the study of patients with photosensitive epilepsy. Their responses to a series of flashes of light are much larger and quite distorted compared with the responses seen in normal people.

The effect of epileptic discharges. Some interesting experiments have been carried out using conventional E E G apparatus, with a view to determining the effect of epileptic discharge on the behaviour of the patient. It was mentioned earlier that epilepsy did not appear to impair the intelligence of the sufferer. However, it is known that a fit itself does affect psychological performance. Clearly a major fit causes unconsciousness, and therefore amnesia. Less is known about the effect of minor attacks or *petit mal*, which were studied by Margerison and Tizard. Essentially, they recorded the EEG and asked the patient to carry out a task at the same time. Then the performance of the patient was related particularly to the length of the electrical disturbance recorded on the EEG.

For this study the patient had electrodes attached to the scalp with glue in the usual way, but was sitting before a table rather than lying on a couch in the usual manner for recording an EEG. A variety of tasks were then given, all rather similar in form. For example, a series of random numbers recorded on tape were played and the patient was asked to press a key every time he heard the number 6. The reaction times during periods when there was or was not epileptic activity in the EEG were examined. Patients were used who showed a particular type of discharge—spike and wave—which is easy to see on the EEG, and the beginning and end of which is easy to decide. Other tasks were used in which the subject had to respond to lights rather than sounds, so that the reaction time to different tasks could also be measured. It was found that the longer the burst of spike and wave, the slower was the reaction time for each task, but quite often patients could work throughout the discharge. There was, however, considerable variation between individuals.

A series of studies by Hutt has also indicated that there is a complex relationship between minor epileptic seizures, the accompanying EEG activity and the task which the person is asked to perform. He has shown with children that it is possible, by changing the difficulty of the task, to arrive at a set of conditions under which the amount of epileptic discharge in the EEG is reduced to a minimum and the performance of the child is optimal. These studies, which have been carried out on a relatively small numbers of patients, have considerable application to the education of children both with epilepsy and other conditions of brain dysfunction. In the long run this may indi-

cate to teachers the best way to help children with such disorders and counteract the reading disability which many of
them show (see below—the work of Rutter and colleagues).

It can be seen that miniaturised E E G apparatus, capable of
transmitting brain activity and attached to the patient's head,
would make it feasible to relate behaviour and electrical activity
even more accurately than was possible in this study of Margerison and Tizard. Such a study, especially in young children who
do not like to be encumbered with apparatus, would be
especially valuable. This applies particularly to hyperkinetic
children who, as a result of some form of brain damage with or
without epilepsy, are markedly over-active. Conventional
E E G recordings in the waking state are impossible for them and
the presence of fits of a minor type can often only be surmised.

Research on temporal lobe epilepsy. As mentioned in chapter III,
confusion arises when the terms temporal lobe attacks and
psychomotor attacks are used. These are both recent names
applied to the attacks described originally at the end of the
nineteenth century by Hughlings Jackson, who coined the term
"dreamy state". In temporal lobe epilepsy, other types of attack
occur as well, and certainly there are various forms of psychomotor fits. Since the advent of the E E G, attempts have been
made to include specific E E G findings with the clinical description of the fit, but this is not entirely helpful in clarifying the
issues. Douglas Northfield, a neuro-surgeon, observed that the
form of epilepsy associated with temporal lobe disorder can
arise with lesions outside the temporal lobe itself.

So that this confused area could be elucidated, Margerison
and colleagues examined several hundred patients to determine
what sort of fit they had. Other witnesses than the patient were
used as far as possible. A neurological examination was carried
out independently of the information already obtained, as well
as detailed special E E G investigations. Then these separate
threads were drawn together. However, a further strand of information was added. The brain from these patients as they
died, from epilepsy or other natural causes unrelated to epilepsy,

was examined by a pathologist, again independently of the other types of information.

As a result of such a careful prospective study, with definite criteria for the diagnosis, it was possible to be certain that all the patients had temporal lobe epilepsy. The pathological findings were, however, very interesting, for they revealed the presence of areas of damaged nerve cells not only in the temporal lobes themselves, but remote from them. These findings would, of course, confirm the earlier quoted observations of Northfield, and in addition indicate the complexity of this form of epilepsy. It may also, to some extent, explain why temporal lobectomy for epilepsy does not produce 100 per cent success. Many problems remain—how did the brain cells become damaged, and why did they produce epileptic discharges? Furthermore, why are there many forms of brain cell damage but only a few which give rise to epilepsy?

Another study in Britain is under the care of Christopher Ounsted and his colleagues at Park Hospital in Oxford. Some of their results have recently been published under the title "Biological factors in temporal lobe epilepsy". A detailed study was carried out on 100 children with temporal lobe epilepsy. The early life of the child, his birth and illnesses in the first years were recorded in detail. The conclusion was reached that infections of the brain (encephalitis) and its coverings (meningitis) were important in the genesis of epileptic fits. Also, about one-third of the children who developed temporal lobe epilepsy had febrile convulsions. This raises the difficult question, did the febrile convulsions damage the brain and lead to fits, or did the child have an epileptic tendency which led to the fits?

Other aspects of temporal lobe epilepsy were investigated by Currie and his colleagues at the London Hospital. A survey of 666 patients with temporal lobe epilepsy was carried out, with a view to determining the different types of fits which each had suffered, as well as attempting to find what was the basis for the temporal lobe disturbance. Was it, for example, a previous head injury, or perhaps convulsions in infancy—a feature which was indeed noted in 5 per cent of the patients? However, the main purpose of the study was to determine the "natural history" of the condition. It was found that 40 per cent of the group were free from attacks for an average of four years and in a further 33 per cent there was a marked reduction both of frequency and severity of fits. As noted in other studies, there is always a proportion of patients in whom treatment with anticonvulsants and other measures fails to lead to satisfactory improvement. In the investigation of Currie 22 per cent had an unchanged frequency of attacks and in 5 per cent there was a distinct increase in the number of fits. Some patients in the series were treated by temporal lobectomy, and this proved to be a useful method of therapy in the cases resistant to medication.

The epidemiological approach. In chapter I it was mentioned that a recent survey of neurological disease had been carried out in Carlisle. This gave definite numbers of patients who suffered from epilepsy and other neurological disorders, such as Parkinsonism and disseminated sclerosis. Such a survey reveals the hidden incidence of disease and shows many problems not obvious to the doctor, whose work is based on the hospital and who waits there for patients to come to him. It has been realised in recent years that, in order to get the accurate incidence of a disease, it is necessary to examine carefully a geographically selected group population and find every single case. This is similar to the approach of the chest physician involved in mass-radiography. The attempt there is to find the "pool of infection" in patients who do not attend their doctors.

A survey in the Isle of Wight organised by Rutter and colleagues was aimed at finding, in a population of school children, the number who were, for example, backward in reading or who had various handicaps. Their particular aim was to delineate the size of the problem so that appropriate services could be provided. A comprehensive examination of a proportion of all the children on the island was carried out over two years, and some of the information is still being analysed. It was found that "compared with the general population of children with chronic physical disorders, not involving the brain, there was a much increased rate of psychiatric disability in children with neuro-epileptic conditions, and this difference was not accounted for in terms of age or sex differences between the groups". This psychiatric disorder appeared to be related specifically to the presence of brain dysfunction. However, they also observed that the cause of psychiatric disorder was the same in the group of neuro-epileptic children as in other groups, that is, factors such as maternal psychiatric illness and "broken homes" lead to a greater incidence of behavioural and psychological disturbance. This detailed study, although it answers some questions, also raises a whole series of others, in particular how best to cope with the educational requirements of these children. It was found, for example, that the neuro-epileptic group of children had considerable reading disability, but the solution of this problem was naturally outside the scope of such an investigation.

The conclusions of Bagley in his statistical study of 118 epileptic children are of interest, and not dissimilar to those of Rutter and colleagues. He observes that "behaviour disorder in epileptic children is the result of the inter-action of a number of factors". Among these he mentions parental attitudes, environmental hazards and brain injury. These are the same factors that lead to disturbance in other children, and there is no specific cause or type of disorder noted in epileptic children.

Another survey, carried out by J. E. Cooper, found that those children with fits who had an obvious illness before the age of two, did less well than expected at school when they began at the age of six. However, when these children were again examined at age 11–15, previous findings were much less marked, and they had in fact almost caught up with their more fortunate fellows. For those interested in the epidemiological approach to epilepsy further studies are included in the bibliography.

Advances in biochemistry. Advances have also been made in the field of human biochemistry, one aspect of which is concerned with chemical examination of the body fluids. This is important in relation to epilepsy. As has already been mentioned, retention of water in the body pre-menstrually and during pregnancy may lead to an increased frequency of epileptic fits. Particularly careful studies are required in which the diet has to be controlled and analysis made of the various body fluids and excretions. This is a complex and time-consuming occupation, but can be of great interest. Dawson and his colleagues published in 1961 a fascinating study of a patient who had defective control of bodily fluids called diabetes insipidus, as well as epilepsy. It was found, if the patient was overhydrated, i.e. had an excess of water, she had more fits, and more epileptic abnormality in her EEG recording. It was actually possible to count the number of spike discharges in the EEG and relate this to the state of hydration of the patient. The reverse was also true. When she was relatively dehydrated she had fewer fits and less spike abnormality on the EEG.

Another type of observation has recently been made on patients with epilepsy, who have for many years been taking anti-convulsants. These patients are sometimes anaemic, and more frequently have levels of circulating vitamins in the blood (Vitamin B_{12} and folic acid) which are well below normal. These observations have been followed by Reynolds and colleagues, who suggest tentatively that this lowering of the vitamin levels is directly related to the action of the anti-convulsant drugs. In addition, it was suggested that these blood changes could be responsible for the rare schizophrenia-like psychosis which has been reported in some epileptic patients (see chapter IX). Neither of these suggestions has been fully proved but they have already sparked off valuable research by other doctors. Incidentally, there has never been any indication that anti-convulsants affect the developing foetus during pregnancy.

Long-term anti-convulsants have been shown to cause yet another type of disturbance. This is in the body chemistry of an important element: calcium. It is essential for a healthy nervous system and in addition is needed for proper development and maintenance of the bony skeleton. Richens and his colleagues have demonstrated, in a detailed study on patients resident in an epileptic colony, that the level of calcium in the blood is decreased and that there is some de-calcification of bones as well. Other disturbances have also been noted: none are specific for one anti-convulsant, but all seem rather to be related to the overall dosage of medications and the length of time for which they have been given. Gross enlargement of the lips and nose has been observed, with thickening of the tissues of the face and scalp, by a group of American doctors (Lefebvre and colleagues) working in a state institution for the mentally retarded.

These recent findings, as well as the unproved suggestion that some anti-convulsants may lead to abnormality in the unborn child, indicate that the existing anti-epileptic medications are by no means perfect, and that the disturbances of the body chemistry and its tissues in general are the price paid for prolonged seizure control. They should stimulate further research and indeed may in the long run give clues to the basic causation of epilepsy itself.

Another aspect of human biochemistry is the investigation of unusual substances sometimes found in the body, for example, copper or lead. It is known that children who chew lead, e.g. from toy soldiers or lead paint, absorb this material from the intestine into the bloodstream. Convulsions may result. Less known is the presence of copper in the blood. A recent study in the journal *Epilepsia* in 1966 suggested that the copper content of the body was lower in patients with epilepsy than those without. This suggestion requires further examination.

A similar biochemical observation started an earlier train of research. In 1952 an observer noticed that children who had by chance been fed on dried milk deficient in vitamin B_6 (a substance known as pyridoxine) developed convulsions. The question was whether these convulsions could be prevented by adding pyridoxine to the diet. As a result of this observation a search was made for other children with fits, who could likewise be treated by pyridoxine. Unfortunately, very few people who have fits suffer from a lack of pyridoxine and respond to treatment in this way. It was a hopeful line of investigation which petered out.

Do we now have any further information about the basic epileptic process itself and how it arises at a cellular level? Hillman, in a recent article on "the chemical basis of epilepsy", put forward a view that the fundamental disturbance is the permeability of the membrane which surrounds the cells in the brain. He thought that the build-up of the element potassium outside cells could spark off their rapid firing, the prelude to fits. Assuming that this could not be suppressed, it would proliferate and lead to a full-blown epileptic attack. He also pointed out that in order to restore the balance of the potassium ions, high energy phosphorus compounds were required. This is at present mere speculation, but animal experiments in which detailed electrical and biochemical data were collected simultaneously could lead to confirmation or refutation of this hypothesis. Meantime we wait for a major breakthrough in the cause and treatment of epilepsy, and try to look after our patients as best we can using the drugs and methods available.

Research on Epilepsy in the United States. Because of the relative ignorance about the causation and treatment of neurological disease in general, and epilepsy in particular, the United States Government set up a vast programme of research in the National Institutes of Health in Washington. In the first instance it was largely a matter of bringing together the basic information about epilepsy and its related subjects. As a result of this campaign a whole series of publications is available to those all over the world interested in epilepsy. A number are listed in the Bibliography, but one volume, *Basic Mechanisms of the Epilepsies*, is of particular importance. In it, world authorities put forward views on the structure and function of the brain, and what happens, and how, in the basic epileptic process. There are also important sections on the actions of anti-convulsants and on animal studies being carried out. Another valuable service was the foundation of "epilepsy abstracts". These contain summaries of all important papers on epilepsy and related matters. However, the U.S. Government programme was concerned not only with the collection of information and its wide dissemination, but also with a multi-disciplinary approach to services for the epileptic patient. Some of these aspects are reported by Cereghinoff and colleagues. After surveying existing services in selected areas of the United States, community service projects were set up. They involved post-graduate education for neurologists, and the training of E E G technicians, neurological nurses and social workers. There was also dissemination of material aimed at the general public, to increase their level of awareness of the problems of the epileptic patient. The benefits of this expensive programme will take many years to accrue and assess, but the fact that this type of programme can be effective has already been shown in the U.S.A. A series of surveys was carried out by Caverness and Merritt in association with the American Institute of Public Opinion to support this view.

The results were surprising and gratifying. A representative group of the population in various areas of the U.S.A. was sampled during the years 1949, 1954, 1959 and again in 1964. The questions asked were, "Would you object to your child playing with a child with epilepsy?"—"Should epileptic patients be employed?" and "Is epilepsy a form of insanity?" In answer to the first question in 1954, 57 per cent said they would not object, while in 1964 the percentage of those who would not object had risen to 77 per cent. With the other two questions there was also a marked reduction of prejudice, but it was still present. The sample represented educated, employed, young urban dwellers who might be less prejudiced than other groups in any case. However, those from the south were more prejudiced than those from either the east or west coasts. Overall, there had been a significant and rewarding change of heart.

Problems in other countries. In *Epilepsia* and *The Candle* (Journal of the British Epilepsy Association) reports have been published in recent years about social problems of epileptics in many countries. In Japan, for example, no Epilepsy Association exists and, though there is low cost treatment for about ten years after diagnosis, the purchase of anti-convulsants can be a costly problem for those with epilepsy. However, in Japan the prevalence of epilepsy is said to be smaller, about 1 in 500 of the population, and not 1 in 200 as in Britain. In addition, there is little prejudice against epilepsy.

In the Netherlands there is a special epilepsy centre at Meer en Bosch, where a diagnostic service and medical treatment is offered, as well as a social rehabilitation centre, a sheltered workshop, a school and facilities for long-term care. This is closely linked with the Evangelical Church and supported by members of an organisation called "the Power of the Small". Members, about 300,000 of them, contribute small sums annually—about 25 to 50 pence. Deacons of the Church are trained as social workers and assist in a chain of out-patient dispensaries in a dozen towns. In this way many people are involved in trying to secure a better understanding of epilepsy.

A country like Nigeria, which is developing rapidly, has very real problems in caring for epileptic sufferers. Epilepsy is more common there than in Europe, and, as primitive medical practices still exist, considerable problems arise, rather like those in earlier times in Europe. Impulsive acts are perpetrated by well-meaning relatives in order to rouse epileptic patients during the fits, and in the sleepy state following them. Those with epilepsy in Nigeria are still labelled as "possessed" and are shunned at school and work.

"People with Epilepsy"

A Government report "People with Epilepsy" was published in Britain in 1969. As mentioned earlier (see p. 128), plans for improved care of epileptic patients put forward by previous Government Committees have had little effect. The recent report, like the earlier, also has excellent recommendations, but their implementation has so far been somewhat limited. Essentially "People with Epilepsy" indicated that the present services for epileptic people were insufficient and recommended the setting up of diagnostic and assessment services in hospitals, particularly those already equipped with neurological and neurosurgical units. The multi-disciplinary approach was recommended, the team consisting not only of the consultant neurologist but also the neurophysiologist and other important ancillary workers such as the clinical psychologist and the social worker. The appropriate local authority staff, including the disablement resettlement officer, would also be involved.

There were to be, in addition, special centres where epileptic people with particular management problems would be considered—six centres in England and Wales in the first instance. Not only would there be the usual neurological and neuro-surgical services, but also a residential unit where detailed assessments of the patient could be carried out. These centres would form focal points for investigation into various aspects of epilepsy as well as for teaching on the subject. All this was considered necessary since it was found that patients often did not have access to the facilities and the treatment they required.

The setting up of special centres and special clinics for epileptic patients is not welcomed by all members of the medical profession, because this could lead to proliferation of services if every diagnostic group were to have its own special facilities. It would mean, for example, clinics for patients with multiple sclerosis and so on. Probably for this reason the report "People with Epilepsy" suggested that existing neurological and neurosurgical and investigatory services should be re-arranged to cope with the special clinics. These should be created, as it were, from existing resources and not involve a great increase in expenditure of money. This was also the recommendation in relation to epileptic patients who required welfare services. These should be provided within the general framework of facilities for the handicapped. In 1972—3 years after the publication of the report and only just following a conference on it run by the Department of Health and Social Security, at which groups of interested people considered the recommendations—it is not possible to indicate what effect the report will have; we must just wait and see.

Social Workers. The report "People with Epilepsy" suggested that social workers can play an important part in the management of patients with seizure disorders, a role which has previously not been fully understood. The social worker may help the man with fits to find a job or obtain suitable lodgings. Although these problems cannot easily be solved, at least he can discuss the difficulties and the social worker can direct him to the appropriate authorities. In this way his personal relationships can be improved and his potential social isolation can be counteracted. The family doctor, to whom the patient may first turn, very often has neither the detailed knowledge nor the time to deal with the social and economic problems of his epileptic patients unaided. He should therefore have recourse to the Social Work Service of the local Health and Welfare Department, where help can be obtained.

The difficulties that parents have with epileptic children and adolescents may also call for the help of a social worker. She may be able to act as a support at times of particular difficulty, and arrange for appropriate services as needed.

It is clear that if the epileptic patient is going to be assisted by social workers at times of crisis then the social workers must be well trained and understand the implications of epileptic brain dysfunction. Similarly, if a teacher is to accept the child with fits in her class without undue tension, she must be aware of the nature of the disorder and its treatment.

Perhaps the biggest hurdle is still prejudice in the community, a prejudice which can be slowly and steadily eroded. In the view of Taylor and Bower, "The efforts which have been made to improve public attitudes to epilepsy have achieved a great deal to lessen its stigma. Yet epilepsy is still surrounded by much mystery and fear. Public enlightenment may not become complete until technical advances prove that man is master of this condition; and this is more likely to be brought about by prevention than cure."

Conclusion

Prejudice against epilepsy and the epileptic sufferer, though it appears to be lessening in the United States, still exists in the world at large. The only effective way of overcoming prejudice and ignorance is through publicity and education. Publicity of the kind that appeared at the time of the Ruby trial can only have deleterious effects. However, education and publicity are not the only aspects of epilepsy that are important in improving the lot of the epileptic person. Solid, reliable, accurate information is perhaps the most important, and this can only be achieved by careful observation and research. This information will be useful for teachers, employers, as well as parents and patients. There is no doubt that honesty on the part of the epileptic patient to friends and employers is best in the long run, and that unnecessary restriction, either self-imposed or imposed by parents, can only lead to further difficulties or resentment. It is important for those who do not suffer from epilepsy to realise the extent of the problem, so that those with epilepsy have a chance in the future to lead a better and fuller life than many have done until now.

Bibliography

THIS contains a list of reference books, medical articles and pamphlets(P). Those particularly suitable for the non-medical reader are marked with an asterisk (*). General references are given first, followed by those in chapter order. Each reference is listed only once under the earliest chapter to which it is applicable. References of interest not directly mentioned in the text have been included.

General†

Barrows, H. S., and Goldensohn, E. S. *Handbook for Parents*. Imperial Chemical Industries Ltd., Cheshire, England (P).
Brain, R. *Paroxysmal and Convulsive Disorders in Diseases of the Nervous System* (6th Edition). Oxford Medical Publications, London (1962).
Grinker, R. R., and Sachs, A. I. *The Epilepsies in Neurology* (6th Edition). Charles, C. Thomas, Springfield, Illinois (1966.)
Lennox, W. G. *Epilepsy and Related Disorders*. Churchill, London (1960).
*Livingstone, S. *Living with epileptic seizures*. Charles C. Thomas, Springfield, Illinois (1963.)
*Pond, D., and Johnson, E. M. *Epilepsy and Fits*. British Medical Association, London (1964) (P).
Pryse-Phillips, W. *Epilepsy*. Wright, Bristol (1969).

CHAPTER II
Bickford, R. G., Whelan, J. L., Klass, D. W., and Corbin, K. B. *Reading Epilepsy*. Trans. Amer. Neurol. Assn. (1956).
Daly, D. D., and Barry, M. J. *Musicogenic Epilepsy: Reports on Three Cases*. Psychosomat. Med. (1957).
Eisner, V., Pauli, L. L., and Livingston, S. *Epilepsy in the Families of Epileptics*. J. Pediat. (1960).
Goldie, L. and Green, D. M. "A study of the psychological factors in a case of sensory reflex epilepsy." *Brain* (1959).

† See also under chapter XVII for recent general references.

Bibliography

"Neurological diseases in Carlisle." *Brit. Med. J.* (1967).
Rowan, A. J., Heathfield, K. W. G., and Scott, D. F. "Is reading epilepsy inherited?" *J. Neurol. Neurosurg. and Psychiat.* (1970).
Servis, et al. "Symposium on reflex mechanisms in the genesis of epilepsy (Prague 1960). *Epilepsia* (1962).
Sherwood, S. I. "Self-induced Epilepsy." *Arch. Neurol.* (1962).
Tower, D. *Neuro-chemistry of Epilepsy: Seizure Mechanisms and their Management.* Charles C. Thomas, Springfield, Illinois, U.S.A. (1960).
Victor, M., and Brausch, C. "The Role of Abstinence in the Genesis of Alcoholic Epilepsy." *Epilepsia* (1967).

CHAPTER III
Ajmone-Marsan, C., and Ralston, B. L. *The Epileptic Seizure – Its Functional Morphology and Diagnostic Significance.* Charles C. Thomas, Springfield, Illinois (1957).

CHAPTER IV
*Grey Walter, W. *The Living Brain.* Duckworth, London (1953, 1961).
Hill, D., and Parr, G. *Electroencephalography.* MacDonald, London (1965).
Kiloh, L. G., and Osselton, J. W. *Clinical Electroencephalography* (2nd edition). Butterworth (1966).
Scott, D. F., and Dodd, B. *Neurological and Neurosurgical Nursing.* Pergamon Press, London (1966).

CHAPTER V
Barolin, G. S. "Migraine and Epilepsies – a relationship." *Epilepsia* (1966).
Gowers, Sir William. *The Borderland of Epilepsy.* P. Blakiston, Son and Co., Philadelphia (1907).
Scott, D. F., Moffett, A., and Swash, M. "Observations on the relation of migraine and epilepsy: an electroencephalographic, psychological and clinical study using oral Tyramine." *Epilepsia* (1972).

CHAPTER VI
Bird, C. A. K., Griffin, B. D., Miklsszeska, J. M., Galbraith. "Tegretol (Carbamazepine): A control trial of a new anticonvulsant." *Brit. J. Psych.* (1966).
Fenton, G. W., Serafetinides, E. A., and Pond, D. A. "The effect of Sulthiame, a new anticonvulsant drug treatment of temporal lobe epilepsy." *Epilepsia* (1964).
Heathfield, K. W. G., and Jewbery, E. C. O. "Treatment of Petit Mal Epilepsy with Ethosuximide." *Brit. Med. J.* (1961).
Hanson, R. A. "Anti-convulsant Drugs." *Practitioner* (1964).
Kutt, H., Winters, W., Scherman, R., and McDowell, F. "Diphenyl-hydantoi and Phenobarbitol toxicity." *Arch. Neurol.* (1964).

174

Liu, M. C. "Clinical experience with sulphiame (ospolot)." *Brit. J. Psychiat.* (1966).

Pryse-Phillips, W. E. M., and Jeavons, P. M. "The effect of carbamazepine (Tegretol) on the electroencephalograph and ward behaviour of patients with chronic epilepsy." *Epilepsia* (1970).

Rowan, A. J., and Scott, D. F. "Major status epilepticus." *Acta. Neurol. Scandinav.* (1970).

CHAPTER VII

Hill, D., Pond, D. A., Mitchell, W., and Falconer, M. A. Personality Changes following temporal lobectomy for Epilepsy." *J. Med. Sci.* (1957).

Meyer, V. "Psychological effects of brain damage." *Handbook of Abnormal Psychology*, ed. H. Eysenck. Pitman Medical, London (1960).

Penfield, E. W. G., and Jasper, H. H. *Epilepsy and the Functional Anatomy of the Brain.* Churchill, London. (1954).

Serafetinides, E. A., and Falconer, M. A. "The effects of temporal lobectomy in epileptic patients with psychosis." *J. Ment. Sci.* (1962).

Taylor, D. T., and Falconer, M. A. "Changes in clinical, socio-economic and psychological adjustment after temporal lobectomy." *Brit. J. Psych.* (1968).

Quadfasel, A. F., and Pruyser, P. "Cognitive deficit in patients with psychomotor epilepsy." *Epilepsia* (1955).

CHAPTER VIII

Jeavons, P. M., and Bower, V. D. *Infantile Spasms.* Clinics in Developmental medicine. No. 15. Medical Education Information Unit, The Spastic Society in association with W. Heinemann Ltd., London (1964).

Keith, H. M. *Convulsive Disorders in Children.* Churchill, London (1963).

Rowan, A. J., and Scott, D. F. "The management of children with epilepsy." *The Practitioner* (1970).

CHAPTER IX

Mayer-Gross, W., Slater, E., and Roth, M. *Clinical Psychiatry* (2nd edn.) Cassell, London (1960).

Pond, D. A. "Psychiatric Aspects of Epilepsy and Brain-damaged children." *Brit. Med. J.* (1961).

Pond, D. A. "Psychiatric Aspects of Epilepsy." *J. Ind. Med. Prof.* (1957).

Slater, E., Baird, A. W., and Glithero, E. "The schizophrenia-like Psychosis of Epilepsy." *Brit. J. Psychiat.* (1963).

Tizard, B. "The Personality of Epileptics. A discussion of evidence." *Psychological Bulletin.* (1962).

CHAPTERS X AND XI

Alajouanine, T. "Dostoewski's Epilepsy." *Brain* (1963).

*Bryant, J. E. *Genius and Epilepsy.* Old Depot Press, Concord, Mass. (1953).

Gowers, W. R., *Epilepsy and other Chronic Convulsive Diseases; their causes, symptoms and treatment*. Dover Publications, New York (1964).

Hemphill, R. E. "The Illness of Vincent van Gogh." *Proc. Roy. Soc. Med.* (1961).

Sieveking, E. H. "Analysis of 52 cases of Epilepsy by the author." *Lancet*, (1857).

Taylor, J. (ed). *Selected Writings of John Hughlings Jackson, Vol. 1*. Hodder and Stoughton (1951).

*Tempkin, O. *The Falling Sickness*. John Hopkins Press, London (1972).

*Wells, C. *Bones, Bodies and Disease*. Thames and Hudson, London (1964.)

CHAPTER XII

Brain, R. *Some Reflections on Genius and other essays*. Pitman Medical, London (1960).

Evans, Margiad. *A Ray of Darkness*. Roy Publishers, New York (1953).

CHAPTER XIII

Alström, C. H. A Study of Epilepsy in its Clinical, Social and Genetic Aspects. *Acta Psychiatrica et Neurologica* (1950). Supplementum 63.

Gunn, J., and Fenton, G. "Epilepsy, automatism and crime." *Lancet* 1. 1173-6.

Fenton, G. W., and Udwin, E. I. "Homicide temporal lobe epilepsy and depression: a case report." *Brit. J. Psychiat.* (1965).

Juul-Jensen, P. "Epilepsy. A clinical and social analysis of 1,020 adult patients with epileptic seizures." *Acta Neurologica Scand.* (1963). Vol. 40, Suppl. 5.

Levin, W. "Epileptic Clouded States: a review of 52 cases." *J. Nerv. Ment. Dis.* (1952).

Scott, P. D. "Medical aspects of delinquency." *Hospital Medicine* (1966).

CHAPTER XIV

Barrow, R. I., and Fabing, H. D. *Epilepsy and the Law*. Hoeber-Harper, New York (1956).

Employing someone with Epilepsy (prepared by Ministry of Labour). Central Office of Information, London (1967) (P).

Epilepsy and Driving Licences (Report of a Symposium in Vienna, September 1965). British Epilepsy Association, International Bureau for Epilepsy. London (1966) (P).

Epilepsy and Employment. British Epilepsy Association and International Bureau for Epilepsy, London (P).

Pond, D. A., and Bidwell, D. M. "A survey of epilepsy in fourteen general practices. II: Social and psychological aspects." *Epilepsia*. (1960).

Total Rehabilitation of Epileptics. U.S. Department of Health, Education and Welfare Office of Vocational Rehabilitation, Washington, D.C. (1962).

Report of the (Cohen) Committee on the Medical Care of Epilepsy. HMSO, London (1956).

CHAPTER XVI

Jennett, W. B. *Epilepsy after Blunt Head Injuries.* Wm. Heinemann Medical Books Ltd., London (1962).

Juul-Jensen, P. "Frequency of Recurrence after Discontinuance of anti-convulsant therapy in patients with epileptic seizures." *Epilepsia* (1964).

Rodin, E. A. *The Prognosis of Patients with Epilepsy.* Springfield, Illinois. Charles C. Thomas (1968).

Taylor, D. C., and Bowyer, B. D. "Prevention of epileptic disorders." *Lancet* (1971).

CHAPTER XVII

Bablouzian, B. L., Neurath, P. W., Sament, S., and Watson, C. W. "Detection of photogenic epilepsy in man by summation of evoked scalp potentials." *Electroenceph. Clin. Neurophysiol.* (1969).

Bagley, C. *The Social Psychology of the Child with Epilepsy.* Routledge and Kegan Paul, London (1971).

Brunia, C. H. M. "Copper Metabolism and Epilepsy." *Epilepsia* (1966).

Caveness, W. F., Merritt, H. H., Gallup, G. H., and Ruby, E. H. "A Survey of public attitudes towards epilepsy in 1964." *Epilepsia* (1965).

Cereghino, J. J., and Cole, C. H. "A multi-disciplinary approach to services for the epileptic." *H.S.M. H. A. Health Reports* April (1971).

Coatsworth, J. J. "Studies on the clinical efficacy of marketed anti-convulsant drugs." N.I.N.D.S. Monograph No. 12. U.S. Department of Health, Education and Welfare. Bethesda, Maryland, U.S.A. (1971).

Cooper, J. E. "Epilepsy in a longitudinal survey of 5,000 children." *Brit. Med. J.* (1965).

Currie, S., Heathfield, K. W. G., Henson, R. A., and Scott, D. F. "Clinical course and prognosis of temporal lobe epilepsy." *Brain* (1971).

Dawson, J., Anderson, W. McC., Margerison, J. H. "Water, electrolytes and the E E G in a case of focal cortical epilepsy with diabetes insipidus on varying drug regimes." *Epilepsia* (1961).

Epilepsy abstracts published monthly by Excerpta Medica Amsterdam, The Netherlands.

Epilepsy in Society. Office of Health Economics. London (1971).

Gastaut et al. "A proposed international classification of epileptic seizures." *Epilepsia* (1964).

Geier, S. "Minor seizures and behaviour." *Electroenceph. Clin. Neurophysiol.* (1971).

Graham, P. J., Rutter, M. L., Yule, W., and Pless, I. B. "Childhood Asthma: a Psychosomatic disorder? Some epidemiological considerations." *Brit. J. Prev. Soc. Med.* (1967).

Gudmundsson, G., "Epilepsy in Iceland." *Acta Neurologica Scand.* (1966). Vol. 43, Suppl. 25.

Hillman, H. "Chemical basis of epilepsy." *Lancet* (1970).

Bibliography

Hutt, S. J. "Experimental analysis of brain activity and behaviour in children with minor seizures." *Epilepsia* (1972).

Jasper, H. H., Wild, A. A. and Pope, A. Editors. *Basic mechanisms of the epilepsies*. J. A. Churchill Limited, London (1969).

Lefebvre, E. B., Haining, R. G., Labbé, R. F. "Coarse facies, calvarial thickening and hyperphosphatasia associated with long term anti-convulsant therapy." *New England Journal of Medicine* (1972).

Margerison, J. H., Corsellis, J. A. N. "Epilepsy and the Temporal Lobes: a clinical, electroencephalographic and neuropathological study of the brain in epilepsy with particular reference to the temporal lobes." *Brain* (1966).

Moffett, A. M., Driver, M. V., St. John Loe, P., Ettlinger, G. "Tactile discrimination performance in the monkey: the effect of unilateral posterior parietal discharging lesions." *Cortex* (1970).

Reynolds, E. H., Chanarin, I., Milner, G., and Matthews, D. M. "Anti-convulsant therapy, folic acid and Vitamin B_{12} metabolism and mental symptoms." *Epilepsia* (1966).

Ounsted, C., Lindsay, J., and Norman, R. *Biological factors in temporal lobe epilepsy*. Clinics in Develop. Med. No. 22. Medical Education and Information Unit. The Spastics Society in association with W. Heinemann Ltd., London (1966).

People with Epilepsy. Department of Health and Social Security. Stationery Office, London (1969).

"Pyridoxine, Tryptophan and epilepsy." *Develop. Med. Child Neurol.* (1965).

Reynolds, E. H. "Schizophrenia-like psychosis of epilepsy and disturbances of folate and Vitamin B_{12} metabolism induced by anti-convulsant drugs." *Brit. J. Psychiat.* (1967).

Richens, A., and Rowe, D. J. F. "Disturbance of calcium metabolism by anti-convulsant drugs." *Brit. Med. J.* (1970).

Rutter, M., Graham, P. and Yule, W. "A neuropsychiatric study in childhood." Clinics in Developmental Medicine, Nos. 35/36. Spastic Medical Publications in association with W. Heinemann. London (1970).

Tizard, B., and Margerison, J. H. "The relationship between generalised paroxysmal E E G discharges and various test situations in two epileptic patients." *J. Neurol. Neurosurg. Psychiat.* (1963).

Wilder, J. B. N.I.N.D.S. Monograph No. 8. U.S. Department of Health, Education and Welfare. Bethesda, Maryland, U.S.A. (1969).

Glossary

Abdominal epilepsy. A condition characterised by periodic abdominal pain and sometimes vomiting. It is thought to be related to epilepsy (see chapter VIII).

Absence. Synonym for *petit mal* (q.v.).

Acidosis. Intoxication of the body by acid substances. This is due to the body's excessively rapid burning-up of oxygen during fits.

Adversive fits. A form of focal epilepsy in which the head and eyes turn to one side and the arms and legs may move on that side also.

Agranulocytosis. An acute illness with ulceration of the throat, mouth and other sites caused by marked reduction of the white blood cells which combat infection; brought about sometimes by antiepileptic drugs.

Air encephalography (also called *Pneumoencephalography*). A special X-ray investigation in which ventricles of the brain are outlined by air.

Akinetic. Sudden weakness of muscles, particularly in the legs.

Alkalosis. Increased alkalinity of the body. One form is brought about by deep breathing during E E G examination.

Amnesia. Loss of memory.

Angiography. A special X-ray investigation in which arteries of the brain are outlined by a contrast medium.

Anti-convulsant. A medication which controls but does not "cure" fits.

Aplastic anaemia. Reduction of red blood cells sometimes due to anti-convulsant medication.

Aphasia. Loss of ability to speak.

Arteriosclerosis. Hardening of the arteries found in middle and old age. See *Cerebral arteriosclerosis.*

Attack. A brief episode which may be epileptic or non-epileptic. In this book there are usually qualifying words, e.g. breath-holding attack, fainting attack, etc.

Aura. A warning of an epileptic attack, e.g. sensation in the abdomen, or a strange smell.

Automatism. Performance of repetitive acts without conscious control. It may occur in the course of a fit or, sometimes, after a major fit.

Glossary

Blackout. Loss of consciousness, sometimes of an epileptic nature; but it may be non-epileptic, e.g. a faint.
Brain storm. A fit of rage, never epileptic in nature.
Brain tumour. A growth in the brain substance. It may be malignant, as in a glioma, or benign, as in a meningioma.
Breath-holding attack. A form of attack following frustration and consequent breath-holding, usually in an infant.

Carotid sinus attack. Over-stimulation of the carotid sinus in the neck, e.g. by a tight collar, when turning the head may lead to a fall in blood pressure and a fainting attack.
Cataplexy. Weakness of the body and limbs, brought on by the expression of emotion, particularly laughter; associated with *Narcolepsy* (q.v.).
Cerebral arteriosclerosis. Hardening of the arteries or vessels of the brain, sometimes causing fits in old age.
Cerebral hemisphere. The upper part of the brain is divided into two masses of nerve tissue, one on the left and the other on the right. Each is a cerebral hemisphere and each is again sub-divided into four regions: the frontal, temporal, parietal and occipital lobes.
Cerebro-spinal fluid. Fluid made in the ventricles of the brain, which escapes through special openings on to the surface and bathes both the brain and spinal cord.
Clonic movements. Rapid to-and-fro jerking movements of the limbs occurring during a major epileptic fit.
Coma. A state of unconsciousness from which the patient cannot be roused, even by painful stimuli.
Convulsion. A violent series of involuntary contractions of muscles; usually associated with complete loss of consciousness.
Cortex. The outer layer of brain tissue consisting mainly of the bodies of the nerve cells.
Craniotomy. An operation in which a section of skull is removed to expose the brain. See also *Trephine.*

Déjà vu. An intense feeling that something has been heard or seen before, even though this is not the case; occurs especially in temporal lobe epilepsy.
Dizziness. Used vaguely to describe a variety of feelings from "light-headedness to a definite rotatory sensation". See also *Vertigo.*
Drop attacks. Attacks in which the person falls suddenly to the ground. These may be epileptic in nature when they occur in young children, but in elderly women, they are usually caused by disease in the arteries at the base of the brain.
Dysrhythmia. An irregular and abnormal pattern of brain rhythm seen in the E E G.

Electrocorticography. Recording of the electrical activity from the exposed cerebral cortex, usually during a neuro-surgical operation.

Electroencephalography. (EEG for short). A recording of the electrical activity of the brain as measured with the aid of electrodes attached to the scalp.

Encephalitis. Inflammation of the brain substance (contrast *Meningitis*).

Epilepsy. Comes from a Greek verb meaning both "to seize" and "to come to a halt". Epilepsy is a repetitive and transient disorder of the brain which leads to fits.

Faint. A brief non-epileptic attack caused by inadequate blood supply to the brain.

Febrile convulsion. A major epileptic attack occurring in infancy during an illness causing fever, e.g. tonsillitis. Sometimes teething fits come into this category.

Fit. A transitory attack, mild or severe. In this book it always means an epileptic phenomenon.

Focal lesion. Area of damaged brain which is the site of origin of epileptic activity.

Focus. An area of brain that is the site of origin of epileptic activity.

Frontal lobe (of the cerebral hemisphere). Concerned particularly with movements of the body and limbs.

Fugue state. A mild disturbance of consciousness lasting from minutes to hours, in which the patient performs purposive acts. May rarely occur after epileptic seizures.

General anaesthetic. A drug or combination of drugs leading to unconsciousness during which a surgical operation can be carried out.

Generalised fit. Disease, etc., not localised or focal, affecting all parts of the brain or body.

Genes. Units of inheritance which transmit from one generation to the next such characteristics as appearance, personality traits and diseases.

Glioma. A cancerous brain tumour.

Grand mal. A major, or convulsive, fit.

Hormone. A substance secreted in the body by an endocrine gland, it has widespread effects on many organs. Some hormones can be used in treatment of diseases such as "infantile spasms".

Hyperkinetic syndrome. A condition in children caused by brain damage, sometimes associated with epilepsy, characterised by marked over-activity and sometimes destructiveness.

Hypnosis. A state of sleep or trance produced by verbal suggestion, used in the treatment of some physical and mental disorders.

Hypocalcaemia. Lowered blood calcium, due to disease, often associated with fits.

Hypoglycaemia. Lowered blood sugar, often due to excessive insulin injection in diabetes.

Glossary

Hypsarrhythmia. An EEG pattern seen in infancy, associated with frequent jerking attacks, an abnormal EEG and sometimes mental subnormality (Synonym—*Infantile spasms*).
Hysteria and *Hysterical attacks.* A neurotic illness characterised by a variety of symptoms which mimic physical disease, including epileptic attacks.

Identical twins. A pair of children conceived after the splitting of a single fertilised ovum, and so sharing the same genetic inheritance. See *Non-identical twins*.
Idiopathic. Condition of unknown cause. A disease not consequent upon any other.
Infantile spasms. A condition characterised by "jack knife" fits (or "salaam attacks") associated with mental subnormality occurring in young infants.

Jacksonian seizure. An attack beginning in a small area of cortex and then becoming more widespread, and sometimes generalised; marked by twitching which may spread along the affected limbs in "marches".
Jamais vu. A temporal lobe attack in which usual surroundings appear strange.

Lesion. Localised injury or disease.
Local. Like "focal", indicates a restriction to one area of the brain or body. Contrast with *Generalised*.
Local anaesthetic. A drug injected into a body tissue to prevent pain locally, so allowing a surgical operation to be carried out without the patient losing consciousness.
Lumbar puncture. A diagnostic test in which a needle is inserted at the base of the spine so that cerebro-spinal fluid (q.v.) may be drawn off for testing.

Major attack. A convulsive attack with a tonic (or rigid) stage followed by a clonic (or jerking) stage. In a major attack there is a complete loss of consciousness (Synonym—*grand mal*).
Meninges. The coverings of the brain and spinal cord.
Meningitis. Inflammation of the meninges.
Mental retardation. A condition due to brain damage or unknown cause in which the person's ability to understand and reason is diminished.
Migraine. A throbbing headache, often one-sided.
Minor attack. Any non-convulsive attack, e.g. *Jacksonian seizure* or *petit mal*.
Myoclonic jerks. Sudden small shock-like jerks of limbs and/or the trunk; may be mild, in association with *petit mal*, or severe enough to throw the patient off balance.

Narcolepsy. A condition characterised by the overpowering desire to sleep. Associated with cataplexy.
Neoplasm. A growth, cancerous or non-cancerous.

182

Nerve. A collection of nerve fibres, grouped in bundles, transmitting impulses from one part of the body to another.
Neuron. A nerve cell, which has a body and an axon, or nerve fibre.
Neuro-surgeon. A brain surgeon.
Neurosis. A mental disorder, usually of mild nature, e.g. anxiety state.
Nocturnal epilepsy. Condition in which attacks occur only at night.
Non-identical twins. Conceived from two separately-fertilised ova. These twins are only as similar in inheritance as in any other two children of the same parents. See *Identical twins.*

Occipital lobe (of the cerebral hemisphere). Located at the back of the head and concerned with processing visual information.

Parietal lobe (of the cerebral hemisphere). Concerned with processing sensory information entering the brain.
Parkinsonism or Parkinson's disease. A chronic disease of the nervous system occurring in middle-aged people, leading to loss of facial expression, rigid muscles and tremors.
Paroxysmal. A condition characterised by periodic attacks. Epilepsy is a paroxysmal condition.
Pathologist. A doctor specialising in the examination of fluids and tissues for diagnosis; often concerned with specimens from dead people to establish the exact cause of death.
Petit mal. A brief epileptic fit, usually occurring in childhood, not associated with convulsive movements but with brief loss of consciousness.
Phenylketonuria. A biochemical disorder of the body, present from birth, causing lowered intelligence and "infantile spasms". An abnormal substance can be detected easily in the urine of the babies affected.
Photic stimulation. Stimulation by flashing lights as in EEG examination.
Pneumoencephalography. See *Air encephalography.*
Prognosis. A forecast of the outcome of a disease or condition.
Psychiatrist. A doctor specially trained to deal with diseases of the mind.
Psychologist. A specialist, usually non medical, in brain and mind function who carries out special tests on humans or animals.
Psychomotor fit. An epileptic attack, characterised by altered awareness, repetitive actions and sometimes amnesia; occurs mainly in *Temporal lobe epilepsy.*
Psychosis. A severe mental disorder, e.g. schizophrenia.
Psychotherapy. A psychological treatment aimed at reducing abnormal emotional responses.
Pyknolepsy. An archaic term for *petit mal* status.

Reflex. A simple action carried out by reflex arc (see chapter II).

Scalp. The skin and muscle layers covering the bones of the head or skull.

Glossary

Seizure. A fit.

Spell. An attack or fit, a term used especially in the U.S.A.

Spike focus. A localised electrical discharge usually in the cortex of the brain, seen on the EEG as a pattern of spikes.

Spike and wave discharge. An electrical disturbance in the brain, usually generalised, associated with fits, especially but not exclusively *petit mal,* and producing on the EEG a characteristic pattern.

Status epilepticus. A serious condition in which one major fit follows another without consciousness being regained.

Stokes-Adams attack. A faint-like attack which results in a sudden fall in the heart rate (due to disease), the brain thereby becoming starved of oxygen.

Stroke. A sudden reduction of blood supply to part of the brain, leading to severe disturbance of function.

Sturge-Weber syndrome. A condition characterised by epilepsy, calcification of the brain and facial birth marks.

Symptomatic. Of known cause (in relation to epilepsy). Contrast with *Idiopathic.*

Syncope. A faint.

Teething fit. See *Febrile convulsion.*

Temper tantrum. An outburst of rage in a child, rarely epileptic in nature.

Temporal lobe (of the cerebral hemisphere). Lying behind the temple: concerned with hearing and memory.

Temporal lobe epilepsy. Fits arising in the temporal lobe, often called psychomotor fits (q.v.). About a fifth of all epileptic attacks are of this kind.

Temporal lobectomy. Surgical removal of part of one temporal lobe sometimes carried out for the treatment of epilepsy.

Tonic. The stage of a major epileptic fit in which muscles of the body are firmly contracted.

Trauma. Injury; particularly when skull is involved, the brain may also be damaged, thus sometimes causing epilepsy.

Tuberous sclerosis. A disease occurring in families, characterised by acne-like condition on the face, calcification of the brain, and convulsions.

Vascular. Of or pertaining to blood vessels. Vascular accident—rupture or blockage of a blood vessel, commonly called a "stroke" (q.v.).

Ventricles. Hollow cavities inside the brain containing the cerebro-spinal fluid which is made there.

Vertigo. A feeling of rotation; giddiness; dizziness.

White matter. The inner layer of brain tissue containing the axons or nerve fibres.

Index